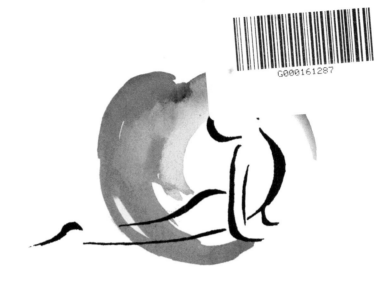

Yogagenda

PLANNER   HANDBOOK   JOURNAL

2O17

My personal info

_____

_____

_____

Founder/Publisher: Elena Sepúlveda - *Yogagenda*

Contributors: Derek Beres, Gary Carter, Bernie Clark, David Ellams, Sattva Giacosa, Lisa Kaley-Isley, Kayla Lakusta, David Lurey, Karen Macklin, Michaela Olexova, Swami Saradananda, Elena Sepúlveda, Michelle Taffe, Carol Trevor, Mirjam Wagner.

Graphic Design: Karoline Leopold

Commissioned Illustrations: Denise Ullmann

Commissioned Photography: Franco Satalino

Front Cover: ©Andrea Haase/Shutterstock.com

Printing: Lighting Source UK/US/Australia Ltd

For more information or to place an order, please visit: **www.YogagendaS.com**

ISBN: 978-0-9572635-3-6

Disclaimer: The publisher, editor and all contributors disclaim any liability or loss in connection with the theories and practices offered in this *Yogagenda*.

Table of Contents

What's in Yogagenda 2017

Namaste and welcome to the current edition of *Yogagenda*. This is our fifth year in print, and to celebrate, instead of five candles, we have chosen five key words to sum up what we have put together to be with you from January to December during 2017. As the months progress and the calendar pages get more and more filled in with your personal entries relating to your life, we'd like to invite you to reflect, heal, create, study, and of course, to practice with us.

Reflect: Why don't New Year's resolutions pan out as intended? Can choosing a yoga teacher training be similar to buying a good breakfast cereal? If you had to focus on one aspect of Pantajali's *Yoga Sutras*, what would that be? What esoteric concepts hide behind seemingly simple yoga stories?

Heal: Yoga has a lot to offer to those within the autism spectrum, and also to people suffering from seasonal sadness. Yoga plus an alkaline diet go a long way to help the body balance itself to its natural healthy state.

Create: Find sound, expert advice for your creative endeavours, whether that is putting together the right playlist for your yoga session, fuelling your writing through meditation practice or setting up a professional yoga blog.

Study: How about exploring the deep anatomy of the foot, the very foundation of our moving structure? What's the common goal of Hatha yoga and acupuncture?

Practice: Discover our *Asana Pages* and this year's Sequence, which together with the Yoga Events and Meditation Centre listings, provide plenty of suggestions for practice.

As usual, within this issue, you will find *Yogagenda*'s fundamental structure with its three distinctive sections: the YEARLY PLANNER, the YOGA HANDBOOK and the JOURNAL PAGES.

We look forward to being with you and supporting your yoga practice throughout the year!

Elena Sepúlveda
Yogagenda Editor
elena@YogagendaS.com

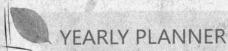

YEARLY PLANNER

We are all about being practical.

This section includes:

- **2 Yearly Calendars** (one for 2017 and another for 2018).

- **1 Closing the Year 2016 - Welcoming the Year 2017** double spread. You may find these pages useful to reflect on the direction your life is taking for the next few months or to recap and plan ahead, as one year comes to an end and the next one begins. As with all of *Yogagenda*'s journal pages, you can be as practical or as reflective as you like!

- **12 Monthly Calendars**, one per page, with space for notes and colour-coded by season.

- **52 Week-at-a-Glance Calendars**, with a week on two pages and colour-coded by season. Weeks are numbered from 1 to 52, and each weekly double spread contains a small month-at-a-glance calendar, plus information on moon phases, solstices, equinoxes and solar/lunar eclipses for 2017. As we are based in Europe, we have adopted a Northern Hemisphere perspective; if you read us from a different part of the planet, please visit www.timeanddate.com for information more relevant to you.

YOGA HANDBOOK

We are all about being informative, and hopefully, inspirational.

All *Yogagenda* contributors are experts in their fields. Coming from different countries and working all over the world, they are practising yoga teachers, living and breathing within the yogic community worldwide. To find out more about them and their work, please go to *Who Contributed to Yogagenda 2017* (pp.242-247).

This section includes:

- **Asana Overview and Asana Pages: Yoga Props to Deepen your Practice.** Illustrated by Denise Ullmann and written by Elena Sepúlveda. Six classic props, each featured twice: first, in a muscularly active type of asana and then in a Restorative yoga asana.

- **Introduction to Restorative Yoga** by Carol Trevor. Find out about this nourishing practice that calms the nervous system by relieving the body and brain of activity and exertion.

- **The Yinside of New Year's Resolutions** by Bernie Clark. New Year's Resolutions tend to be yang in nature, because they are about changing ourselves and our lives. But what about the yin aspects of such intentions?

- **Yoga for Seasonal Sadness** by Lisa Kaley-Isley. The absence of external light in winter may bring about seasonal sadness. Specific yoga techniques can alleviate this problem by connecting us to our essential internal light.

- **Keep Alkaline, Keep Healthy** by Elena Sepulveda. Our diets, mind states and environments are as much allies as challenges for keeping that crucial-for-health balance of acidity and akalinity in our body tissues.

- **Hatha Yoga: the Yang to Acupuncture's Yin** by Kayla Lakusta. Bringing the body into one balanced state of yin and yang is the aim of both acupuncture and yoga, something that can be seen inquiring into one fundamental yoga asana: Tadasana (Mountain Pose).

- **The Science of Movement and Music** by Derek Beres. Silence is definitively preferable to the wrong music being played in a yoga class. Learn some useful facts to make better choices when building playlists for your yoga sessions.

- **Conscious Choices for Teacher Training** by Mirjam Wagner and David Lurey. What do you look for in a yoga teacher training course? The offers can be daunting! Make your choice a conscious one with these simple but well-thought and clear suggestions.

- **Foot, Fascia, Spine: The Spring in our Step** by Gary Carter. Human postural control is a complex process of balancing the motions of all structures of the body in the field of gravity; the very foundation of our moving structure can be considered to come from the foot and the spine.

- **Yoga for Autism** by David Ellams. Yoga4Autism helps people with special needs through the use of healthy natural methods such as yoga and meditation to address causes, rather than cover up symptoms with mind-numbing drugs.

- **Begin Again. And Again. How Meditation Can Support your Artistic Practice** by Karen Macklin. Even if you consider yourself a natural born artist, creative work can test your body, mind and heart. Find out four ways meditation can fuel your creative efforts.

- **10 Expert Tips to Creating a Yoga Blog from Your Heart** by Michaela Olexova. If you feel the urge to express yourself, share and inspire others, blogging can be the best creative platform to you reach your tribe, wherever they are.

- **Renewing Wisdom: Pantajali and the *Yoga Sutras*** by Sattva Giacosa. When it comes to the *Yoga Sutras* and Patanjali, there is one fundamental aspect we can focus on understanding that will draw us nearer to our innate nature.

- **Yoga Teaching Stories** by Swami Saradananda. What better way to understand yoga philosophy than to hear a story that illustrates an esoteric concept? The ancient rishis understood this and made use of the transformative power of teaching stories.

- **Yoga Events and Meditation Centres around the Globe.** Michelle Taffe of the Global Yogi brings us her well-researched listing of yoga events around the world for 2017. This year the listing includes 12 recommended international meditation centres.

- **Sanskrit Glossary.** These pages offer short explanations of the Sanskrit terms used in this edition of *Yogagenda*.

- **Asana Index.** A quick way to find the poses included in the *Asana Pages*.

- **The Sequence: Restorative Yoga to Ease Anxiety** by Carol Trevor. Focussing on creating calm and ease through the experience of rooting and connecting to the earth, this sequence provides stability and containment for the body while gently encouraging a comfortable amount of opening in areas that can feel constrained.

JOURNAL PAGES

We are all about encouraging creative reflection.

This section includes:

- 12 Monthly Change-Accept-Discover Pages. Drawing from the idea introduced in the January article (*The Yinside of New Year's Resolutions*), we have included a journal page per month to explore the dance of yin and yang in goal-setting. These pages provide space to record what you want to change/accomplish, but also to acknowledge what you wish to embrace/accept each month. A third section below allows you to write down any insights or discoveries that may come up from this process.

- My Notes. Each Asana Page and monthly article incorporates space for personal notes relating to these contents.

- Blank Journal Pages at the beginning of each month and the end of *Yogagenda*. These are blank sheets for your own needs: to plan, to journal, to spread your creative wings on paper or for whatever takes your fancy.

Closing the Year 2016

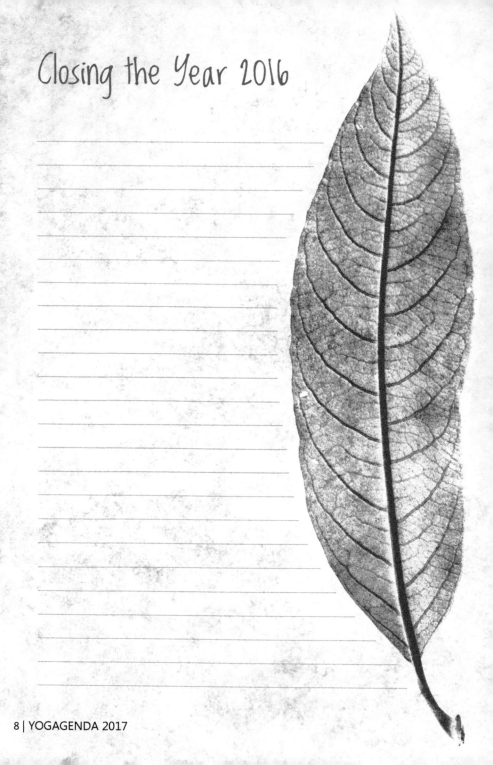

_____

_____

_____

_____

_____

_____

_____

_____

_____

_____

_____

_____

_____

_____

_____

_____

_____

_____

_____

_____

_____

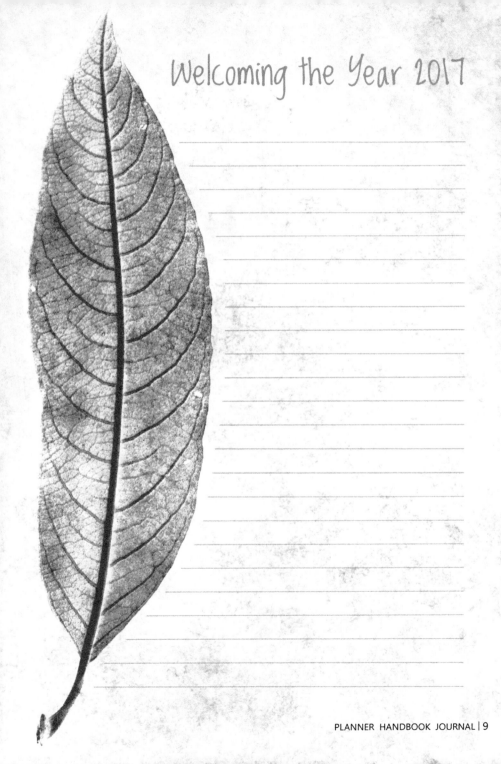

Welcoming the Year 2017

2017

January

						1
2	3	4	5	6	7	8
9	10	11	12	13	14	15
16	17	18	19	20	21	22
23	24	25	26	27	28	29
30	31					

February

		1	2	3	4	5
6	7	8	9	10	11	12
13	14	15	16	17	18	19
20	21	22	23	24	25	26
27	28					

March

		1	2	3	4	5
6	7	8	9	10	11	12
13	14	15	16	17	18	19
20	21	22	23	24	25	26
27	28	29	30	31		

April

					1	2
3	4	5	6	7	8	9
10	11	12	13	14	15	16
17	18	19	20	21	22	23
24	25	26	27	28	29	30

May

1	2	3	4	5	6	7
8	9	10	11	12	13	14
15	16	17	18	19	20	21
22	23	24	25	26	27	28
29	30	31				

June

			1	2	3	4
5	6	7	8	9	10	11
12	13	14	15	16	17	18
19	20	21	22	23	24	25
26	27	28	29	30		

July

					1	2
3	4	5	6	7	8	9
10	11	12	13	14	15	16
17	18	19	20	21	22	23
24	25	26	27	28	29	30
31						

August

1	2	3	4	5	6	
7	8	9	10	11	12	13
14	15	16	17	18	19	20
21	22	23	24	25	26	27
28	29	30	31			

September

				1	2	3
4	5	6	7	8	9	10
11	12	13	14	15	16	17
18	19	20	21	22	23	24
25	26	27	28	29	30	

October

						1
2	3	4	5	6	7	8
9	10	11	12	13	14	15
16	17	18	19	20	21	22
23	24	25	26	27	28	29
30	31					

November

		1	2	3	4	5
6	7	8	9	10	11	12
13	14	15	16	17	18	19
20	21	22	23	24	25	26
27	28	29	30			

December

				1	2	3
4	5	6	7	8	9	10
11	12	13	14	15	16	17
18	19	20	21	22	23	24
25	26	27	28	29	30	31

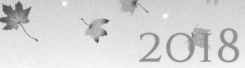
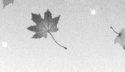

2018

January

1	2	3	4	5	6	7
8	9	10	11	12	13	14
15	16	17	18	19	20	21
22	23	24	25	26	27	28
29	30	31				

February

			1	2	3	4
5	6	7	8	9	10	11
12	13	14	15	16	17	18
19	20	21	22	23	24	25
26	27	28				

March

			1	2	3	4
5	6	7	8	9	10	11
12	13	14	15	16	17	18
19	20	21	22	23	24	25
26	27	28	29	30	31	

April

						1
2	3	4	5	6	7	8
9	10	11	12	13	14	15
16	17	18	19	20	21	22
23	24	25	26	27	28	29
30						

May

1	2	3	4	5	6	
7	8	9	10	11	12	13
14	15	16	17	18	19	20
21	22	23	24	25	26	27
28	29	30	31			

June

				1	2	3
4	5	6	7	8	9	10
11	12	13	14	15	16	17
18	19	20	21	22	23	24
25	26	27	28	29	30	

July

						1
2	3	4	5	6	7	8
9	10	11	12	13	14	15
16	17	18	19	20	21	22
23	24	25	26	27	28	29
30	31					

August

		1	2	3	4	5
6	7	8	9	10	11	12
13	14	15	16	17	18	19
20	21	22	23	24	25	26
27	28	29	30	31		

September

					1	2
3	4	5	6	7	8	9
10	11	12	13	14	15	16
17	18	19	20	21	22	23
24	25	26	27	28	29	30

October

1	2	3	4	5	6	7
8	9	10	11	12	13	14
15	16	17	18	19	20	21
22	23	24	25	26	27	28
29	30	31				

November

			1	2	3	4
5	6	7	8	9	10	11
12	13	14	15	16	17	18
19	20	21	22	23	24	25
26	27	28	29	30		

December

					1	2
3	4	5	6	7	8	9
10	11	12	13	14	15	16
17	18	19	20	21	22	23
24	25	26	27	28	29	30
31						

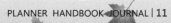

January 2017

Monday	Tuesday	Wednesday	Thursday	Friday	Saturday	Sunday
						1
2	3	4	☽ 5	6	7	8
9	10	11	○ 12	13	14	15
16	17	18	☾ 19	20	21	22
23	24	25	26	27	◐ 28	29
30	31					

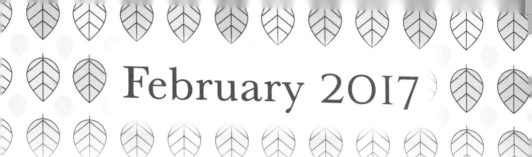

February 2017

Monday	Tuesday	Wednesday	Thursday	Friday	Saturday	Sunday
		1	2	3	◖ 4	5
6	7	8	9	10 Penumbral Lunar Eclipse	○ 11 Penumbral Lunar Eclipse	12
13	14	15	16	17	◐ 18	19
20	21	22	23	24	25	◓ 26 Solar Anular Eclipse
27	28					

March 2017

Monday	Tuesday	Wednesday	Thursday	Friday	Saturday	Sunday
		1	2	3	4	◗ 5
6	7	8	9	10	11	○ 12
13	14	15	16	17	18	19
◖ 20 Spring Equinox	21	22	23	24	25	26
27	○ 28	29	30	31		

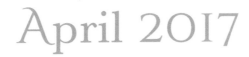

April 2017

Monday	Tuesday	Wednesday	Thursday	Friday	Saturday	Sunday
					1	2
☽ 3	4	5	6	7	8	9
10	○ 11	12	13	14	15	16
17	18	☾ 19	20	21	22	23
24	25	○ 26	27	28	29	30

May 2017

Monday	Tuesday	Wednesday	Thursday	Friday	Saturday	Sunday
1	2	3 ☽	4	5	6	7
8	9	10 ○	11	12	13	14
15	16	17	18	19 ☾	20	21
22	23	24	25 ○ Super New Moon	26	27	28
29	30	31				

June 2017

Monday	Tuesday	Wednesday	Thursday	Friday	Saturday	Sunday
			☽ 1	2	3	4
5	6	7	8	○ 9 Micro Full Moon	10	11
12	13	14	15	16	☾ 17	18
19	20	21 Summer Solstice	22	23	○ 24 Super New Moon	25
26	27	28	29	30		

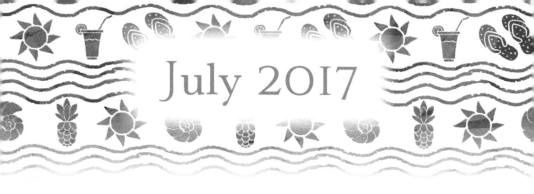

July 2017

Monday	Tuesday	Wednesday	Thursday	Friday	Saturday	Sunday
					◗ 1	2
3	4	5	6	7	8	○ 9
10	11	12	13	14	15	◑ 16
17	18	19	20	21	22	○ 23
24	25	26	27	28	29	◗ 30
31						

August 2017

Monday	Tuesday	Wednesday	Thursday	Friday	Saturday	Sunday
	1	2	3	4	5	6
○ 7 Penumbral Lunar Eclipse	8 Penumbral Lunar Eclipse	9	10	11	12	13
14	◐ 15	16	17	18	19	20
○ 21 Black Moon	22	23	24	25	26	27
28	◑ 29	30	31			

September 2017

Monday	Tuesday	Wednesday	Thursday	Friday	Saturday	Sunday
				1	2	3
4	5	○ 6	7	8	9	10
11	12	☽ 13	14	15	16	17
18	19	● 20	21	22 Autumn Equinox	23	24
25	26	27	☾ 28	29	30	

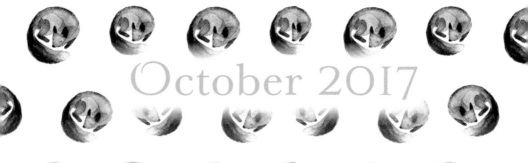

October 2017

Monday	Tuesday	Wednesday	Thursday	Friday	Saturday	Sunday
						1
2	3	4	○ 5	6	7	8
9	10	11	◑ 12	13	14	15
16	17	18	○ 19	20	21	22
23	24	25	26	27	◐ 28	29
30	31					

November 2017

Monday	Tuesday	Wednesday	Thursday	Friday	Saturday	Sunday
		1	2	3	○ 4	5
6	7	8	9	☽ 10	11	12
13	14	15	16	17	● 18	19
20	21	22	23	24	25	☾ 26
27	28	29	30			

December 2017

Monday	Tuesday	Wednesday	Thursday	Friday	Saturday	Sunday
				1	2	○ 3 Super Full Moon
4	5	6	7	8	9	◐ 10
11	12	13	14	15	16	17
○ 18 Micro New Moon	19	20	21 Winter Solstice	22	23	24
25	◑ 26	27	28	29	30	31

Asana Overview - Yoga Props to Deepen Your Practice

By Elena Sepúlveda

The use of props has come to be associated with specific styles of yoga. However, using props can benefit everyone across schools, from beginners to more experienced practitioners, from the injured to the strongest, and the least to the most flexible. Props offer stability and support, enable alignment, encourage flexibility, and provide freedom to explore different aspects of an asana.

In this edition of *Yogagenda*, you'll find six classic props, each featured twice: first in a muscularly active type of asana and then in a Restorative one. Each one of the Asana Pages includes two further suggested props for the featured asana.

All Restorative poses come together in this year's sequence: Restorative Yoga to Ease Anxiety (p.230). Pages 26-27 include an *Introduction to Restorative Yoga* by Carol Trevor.

The featured asanas are:

Salamba Sarvangasana (Supported Shoulderstand) with blanket - pp.44-45.

Balasana (Child's Pose) with blanket - pp.60-61.

Chaturanga Dandasana (Four Limbed Staff Pose or Plank Pose) with bolster - pp.78-79.

Resting Bharadvajasana (Bharadvaja's Pose) Twist with bolster - pp.94-95.

Parivrtta Parsvakonasana (Revolved Side Angle Pose) with block - pp.110-111.

Upavistha Konasana (Wide Angle Seated Forward Bend) with block - pp.128-129.

Janushirsasana (Head to Knee Pose) with belt - pp.144-145.

Setubandha Sarvangasana (Supported Bridge Pose) with belt - pp.162-163.

Viparita Dandasana (Upward Facing Two Foot Staff Pose) with chair - pp.178-179.

Viparita Karani (Legs Up the Wall Pose) with chair - pp.194-195.

Sukhasana (Easy Pose) with cushion - pp.212-213.

Savasana (Corpse Pose) with cushion - pp.228-229.

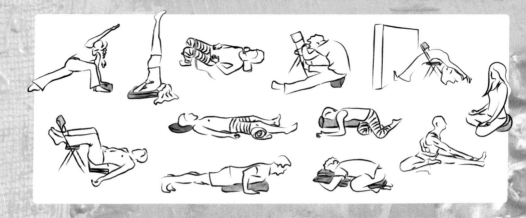

Featured Yoga Props

Blankets

They can be used for elevation or cushioning. Carefully folded or rolled, blankets can support chest openers, forwards bends, inversions and twists. And of course, they are useful to cover yourself during Savanana (Corpse Pose) at the end of a session!

Blocks

Made of cork or foam, blocks add height or length to the body in standing poses, bringing the floor to you. They provide three different heights, depending on whether they are laid flat, placed on edge, or stood on end. In seated poses, they can take the edge off your hamstrings and lower back.

Belts

They encourage flexibility and help deepen stretches when tension in the tissues limits a pose. At the same time, belts provide stability to joints and protect them in case of hyper-mobility. Like all props, belts can help you stay longer in an asana and feel it where it's meant to be felt.

Bolsters

They are helpful to open, release and support a specific part of the body. In Restorative yoga, they elevate the body in inversions and support the limbs and torso. Whether rectangular or cylindrical, they can effectively prop you up during deep spinal stretches.

Chairs

They offer support, adding intensity to rotation in twists and increasing openness in backbends. Chairs can grant better alignment with less effort and extend the range and duration of a pose. Whichever type of chair you use, it's important it is stable and doesn't tip over while doing yoga.

Cushions

Perhaps the most versatile of all yoga props, cushions often take the place of bolsters, blankets, blocks or chairs, but obviously not when a firm, hard surface is needed! In more passive yoga poses, you can relax on the cushion and let gravity and the breath do the asana for you.

Introduction to Restorative Yoga

By Carol Trevor

Restorative yoga is a nourishing practice characterised by its effortlessness and ease. This is created by using props to support the body completely. Poses, including forward and backbends, twists and inversions, are comfortably and passively experienced for some minutes. The cornerstone of the practice is Savasana (Corpse Pose). It is the perfect practice in stressful and busy times.

Restorative yoga calms the nervous system by relieving the body and brain of activity and exertion. We experience deep rest and rejuvenation as layers of tension and tightness are gently released on all levels–physical, mental, and emotional. As such, the practice can also be applied to improve flexibility and overall ease in the body.

By providing access to the parasympathetic branch of the nervous system, Restorative yoga enables us to shift from our active fight-or-flight stress response to our receptive rest-and-digest mode. Our organs and involuntary functions, including heart rate, breathing, digestion, and elimination, then function at their best. On a subtle level, prana–our breath, energy, and life force–flows freely.

Restorative yoga offers a foundation for meditation as our awareness is heightened in the poses. We feel poses in a profound way. The stillness and internal focus reflect pratyahara, one of Patajanjali's eight limbs of yoga, in which we are aware of everything around us, but are not disturbed or dominated by it. We develop the skill of witnessing. In everyday life, this translates into clarity, ease, and emotional balance.

The practice has its roots in the therapeutic work of B.K.S. Iyengar. In Restorative yoga, comfort is key, and many of the props are soft, such as bolsters, blankets, eye pillows and cushions. Blocks and belts contribute to stability and containment and also protect against hypermobility.

Given its direct link with the relaxation response, Restorative yoga is highly beneficial for stress-related conditions, such as insomnia, digestive ailments, tension headaches, non-specific lower back pain, shallow breathing, and anxiety.

Turn to p.230 to see a Restorative sequence to help with anxiety specifically.

Restorative Yoga Props

Yoga Mat

Non-slip.

Yoga Bolster

A firm, cotton-filled cylindrical cushion. Or a rolled-up, firm blanket. Used to lie on, elevate the body in inversions and support the limbs and torso.

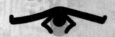

Blankets

Firm, wool or cotton. Or bath towels. Used to soften edges, modify the degree of elevation, extension, or flexion and to provide a sense of security, cosiness and warmth.

Cushions

Medium-sized. Or pillows. Used to support the limbs and head and to modify poses.

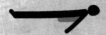

Small Towel

Hand towel. Or cloth, scarf. Used to support the neck, wrists and ankles. Can be placed on the forehead in supine poses to help calm the mind.

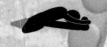

Eye Pillow

Or small folded towel. Placed over the eyes or on the forehead to dissipate mental fluctuations and calm the mind, or in each hand in supine poses to provide a sense of grounding.

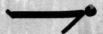

Belt

Yoga belt. Or neck ties. Used to gently bind the feet or limbs to provide containment, relieve the muscles of work and guard against hypermobility.

Weights

5kg and 2kg. Or packs of dry pulses, rice or sugar. Placed, for example, on the lower back or feet for a sense of grounding and to relieve tension. Small weights, such as tea-light candle holders, can be placed in the palms of the hands in supine poses for the same purpose.

Crepe Bandage

Wrapped around the head from its base at the back and covering the ears. In Savasana, this provides deep calm, quieting the mind and minimising the impact of external distractions.

Some poses are done with the support of a wall, chair or table.

The Yinside
of New Year's Resolutions

By Bernie Clark

Chances are you have made at least one New
Year's resolution before. Think back over a few.
Were they about changing something about
yourself? Was there something that you were
doing that you wanted to stop, or something
that you were not doing that you vowed to start?

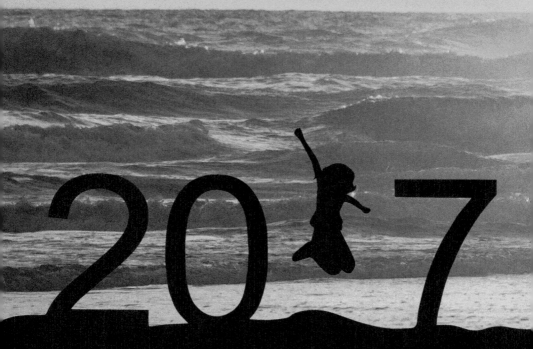

New Year's resolutions are yang in nature and relate to activities: resolving to do or refrain from doing something, or in other words, to change yourself or your life in some way. These can be wonderful intentions, and there are times, not necessarily only on January 1st, when we do need to tap into our yang energies and change the course of our lives. However, to be balanced, we also need to look at the yin aspects of such intentions.

When we examine our resolutions, we find that they are based on the unspoken assumption that the way we are right now is not good enough. There is a *"should"* lurking in our self-evaluation: we should be better–different than we are right now.

Where is that assumption coming from? Why are you not content with the way you and your life are right now?

Whose voice is whispering in your ear that you should be different?

Balance requires consciously honouring both the yin and yang energies of life. Yang is about change, movement, climbing great heights, and accomplishing great deeds. Yin is about acceptance, allowing, enjoying the present moment, and doing small, everyday tasks as if they were great deeds.

In our society and culture, we are constantly urged to change, to improve, to seek what we don't have, and to fix the problems we do have.

It is easy to fall into the belief that however we are right now is inadequate in so many ways. And, since we are so flawed, why not vow to improve? All we need to do is buy certain products, dress in a different way, or change jobs, relationships, locale, etc.

Over the past many years, we may have done all of this and more—and yet, somehow, still feel inadequate. It is easy to blame ourselves for this failure, and that blame just feeds into the next cycle of change: we need to try harder or do more. It is not a surprise that so many New Year's resolutions lie broken and forgotten before the Christmas tree is taken away.

Let's look at the yinside of all of this. What is there about yourself that you can simply accept and not try to change? After all these years of trying to change, select something that you will simply allow to just be.

This is not easy! It is counter-cultural and counterintuitive. Some examples could be:

"I resolve to accept my body just as it is right now!"

"I resolve to allow my anger/fear/depression to manifest without judgement."

"I resolve to stay with my current partner/job/apartment/car/cat..."

"I resolve to let ... (fill in the blank) ... just be."

Perhaps in years past, you resolved to give up something, to lose weight, to stop eating desserts, or to give up chocolate (gasp!). The shadow side of that yang decision may have been losing joy and comfort as you deliberately restricted the amount of pleasure you allowed yourself. As a consequence, you were unhappy, and this unhappiness spread to the loved ones in your life.

This is not to say that these yang resolutions were unwise, but rather to point out that every decision and action has a consequence to it. The key question to ask yourself is, "Am I better having made these resolutions in the past?" It is up to you to define better - healthier, happier, more content, more balanced. If you do not believe you are better off, then it is time to revisit the intention behind your resolutions.

This year, why not resolve to accept something about yourself that you will no longer try to change or improve? Sure, go ahead and consciously make a yang resolution to do or not do something, but why not add a yin resolution this time? What are you going to accept, allow and no longer try to change this year?

Let this year be your year of yin.

my notes

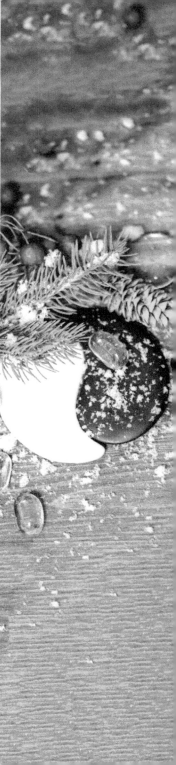

This month I will change

This month I will accept

This month I discovered

January 2017

January 2017

						1
2	3	4	5	6	7	8
9	10	11	12	13	14	15
16	17	18	19	20	21	22
23	24	25	26	27	28	29
30	31					

December 2016 / January 2017

26
MONDAY

27
TUESDAY

28
WEDNESDAY

New Moon ⬤ **29**
THURSDAY

30
FRIDAY

31
SATURDAY

1
SUNDAY

January 2017

						1	week 52
2	3	4	5	6	7	8	
9	10	11	12	13	14	15	
16	17	18	19	20	21	22	
23	24	25	26	27	28	29	
30	31						

January 2017

2
MONDAY

3
TUESDAY

4
WEDNESDAY

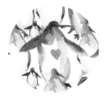

First Quarter ☽

5
THURSDAY

6
FRIDAY

7
SATURDAY

8
SUNDAY

January 2017

						1	
2	3	4	5	6	7	8	week 1
9	10	11	12	13	14	15	
16	17	18	19	20	21	22	
23	24	25	26	27	28	29	
30	31						

9
MONDAY

10
TUESDAY

11
WEDNESDAY

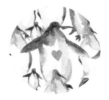

Full Moon ◯ **12**
THURSDAY

13
FRIDAY

14
SATURDAY

15
SUNDAY

January 2017

						1
2	3	4	5	6	7	8
9	10	11	12	13	14	15
16	17	18	19	20	21	22
23	24	25	26	27	28	29
30	31					

week 2

16
MONDAY

17
TUESDAY

18
WEDNESDAY

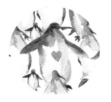

Last Quarter ☾ **19**
THURSDAY

20
FRIDAY

21
SATURDAY

22
SUNDAY

January 2017

						1
2	3	4	5	6	7	8
9	10	11	12	13	14	15
16	17	18	19	20	21	22
23	24	25	26	27	28	29
30	31					

week 3

23
MONDAY

24
TUESDAY

25
WEDNESDAY

26
THURSDAY

27
FRIDAY

New Moon 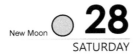 **28**
SATURDAY

29
SUNDAY

January 2017

						1
2	3	4	5	6	7	8
9	10	11	12	13	14	15
16	17	18	19	20	21	22
23	24	25	26	27	28	29
30	31					

week 4

Salamba Sarvangasana

Supported Shoulderstand

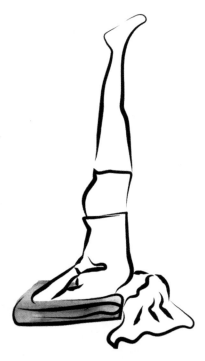

Coming into the Pose

- Place two or three carefully folded blankets on the floor. Keep the edges together and the folded parts smooth, making sure there are no creases.
- Lie on the blanket with your arms and shoulders on it and your head on the floor. Bring your arms close to your torso.
- Bend your legs with your feet close to your buttocks.
- Place your elbows on the floor.
- On an exhale, lift your trunk, bend your legs towards your abdomen and support your back with your hands.
- Raise your trunk and legs higher, bringing your chest towards your chin.
- On an inhale, straighten your legs.
- Bring your elbows towards each other, drawing your shoulder blades in.

While in the Pose

- Tuck your coccyx in.
- Keep the weight on your arms, not your neck.
- Walk your hands up your back to lift further.
- Relax your eyes, forehead and throat.

Coming out of the Pose

Go on to Halasana (Plough Pose) taking your legs to the floor over your head. Otherwise, lower your legs over your head to a 45-degree angle, exhale and slide down carefully vertebra by vertebra, releasing your hands. Once on the floor, go into Apanasana (Knees to Chest Pose) hugging your knees to your chest.

What the Prop Does for the Pose

It helps protect the neck by reducing the amount it has to flex to achieve the pose.

Benefits

- Relaxes the legs and improves blood circulation.
- Nourishes the thyroid and parathyroid glands with blood.
- Improves digestion.
- Alleviates laziness and mental lethargy.

Contraindications

- Neck injuries.
- High blood pressure.
- Glaucoma, headaches.
- Some traditions advise against this pose during menstruation and/or pregnancy.

Other Props for this Pose

Belt. Using a belt around your upper arms brings your shoulder blades towards each other and aids balance.

Chair. Here your back is supported and arched and your chest opens up, allowing your internal organs to stretch.

For full instructions on these poses, check our blog *www.yogagendas.com/blog* each month during 2017.

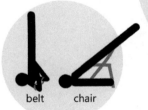

belt   chair

my notes

Yoga for Seasonal Sadness

By Lisa Kaley-Isley

In winter, the absence of external light, together with the urge to keep an unnaturally fast pace for the season may bring about seasonal sadness. Yoga reminds us that "Light is our essence" and offers us techniques to reconnect with our internal light, making it shine stronger so we can see beyond our limiting beliefs and step into self-transformation.

Our senses draw us to experience life. They are the tangible means through which we interact and feel ourselves connected to everything else. We experience everything along the continuum of pleasure and pain, like and dislike in our bodies, minds, and the external world through our senses.

In the yoga tradition, it is said that the unchanging, all knowing Purusha took the form of a body in order to have experience.
It is the yogic answer to "Why did the chicken cross the road?" Answer: to have the experience of crossing the road. It is that vital to us.

For most of us, the majority of the time, the antenaes of our senses are turned outward to gather information from the world around us. Pratyahara, the fifth of the eight limbs of raja yoga, is the reversal of this process: turning the senses inward and shifting the object of attention back to that part of ourselves which is having the experience; consciousness itself. It is a self-reflective process of looking outward to experience, and then looking inward to remember who it is that is experiencing.

The winter months are challenging for many of us because what we see and feel is grey, dark, cold, and wet. It is the seasonal equivalent of the fifth limb and of the daily need to sleep. Winter strongly encourages us to draw inward, rest, and seek warmth and light inside. In the winter, nature takes a break from producing, and when our labours were in sync with the seasons our activities shifted, too.

Now in our modern same-all-year jobs, the vocational demands are the same, but the internal and seasonal cues prompt us to slow and change. This can lead us to feel that the usual activities require greater than normal effort. It's natural to want to sleep longer, curl up someplace warm, light a fire or candle, and hang artificial lights in the trees, streets, and our houses. We have found ways to supplement the external light, but that does not mean we have found a way to reconnect to our inner light and keep it strong when there is not as much sun.

When in the absence of external light we cannot experience our internal light, a seasonal sadness can take hold. Light is our essence, and it is the vehicle of perception. Light is the controller of our daily rhythms and physiological processes. When nature turns down the light, we are affected. It's not just experience we need; we need experience of light. When it runs low, our vitality, mood, and self-concept do, too.

The *Yoga Sutras** say very little about asana, but they describe several pranayama and meditation practices. This how-to manual really focuses on making our internal light so strong that we can see ourselves again.

Sutras 1.34 and 1.35 describe vigorous pranayama practices, and as a result, Sutra 1.36 tells us that an inner light dawns that floods us with illumination.

In the light, we see clearly and are beyond all sorrow. Everything is changed because we can tolerate seeing our everyday foibles and feelings if we know we are not really limited to being them. This self-transformation is the goal and result of enlightenment/becoming lit from within.

Knowing how vital it is to our well-being, make the commitment to connect to light for some period of time every day, especially in the winter. A useful meditation practice is trataka or candle gazing. Sit about 3 feet from the candle so your downward gaze can easily rest on the flame. Keep your eyes open for longer and longer periods of time between blinks. Your eyes may water.

Keep directing your attention to the dancing flame so that it is all you see. Let every other thought go save seeing the light. When you feel the connection firmly established, close your eyes and see if you can now see the flame in your eyebrow centre. If yes, rest there and add silent repetition of the mantra *Om Joytir Ahum*, I am the light beyond all sorrow.

If you cannot yet see the light inside, simply open your eyes and focus again on the flame. Let your sensory perception of visible light reconnect you to your internal light. Follow nature's cues to look inward using the tools to help you connect, and gradually the sadness will lift.

*For more on the *Yoga Sutras* see *The Secret of the Yoga Sutra* by Pandit Rajmani Tigunait, PhD

my notes

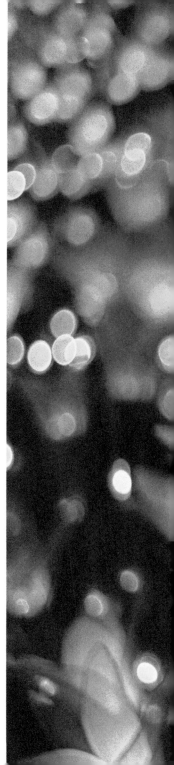

This month I will change

This month I will accept

This month I discovered

February 2017

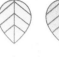

JOURNAL

February 2017

		1	2	3	4	5
6	7	8	9	10	11	12
13	14	15	16	17	18	19
20	21	22	23	24	25	26
27	28					

30
MONDAY

31
TUESDAY

1
WEDNESDAY

2
THURSDAY

3
FRIDAY

First Quarter ◗ **4**
SATURDAY

5
SUNDAY

February 2017

		1	2	3	4	5
6	7	8	9	10	11	12
13	14	15	16	17	18	19
20	21	22	23	24	25	26
27	28					

week 5

6
MONDAY

7
TUESDAY

8
WEDNESDAY

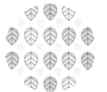

9
THURSDAY

10
Penumbral Lunar Eclipse FRIDAY

Full Moon ◯ **11**
Penumbral Lunar Eclipse **SATURDAY**

12
SUNDAY

February 2017

		1	2	3	4	5	
6	7	8	9	10	11	12	week 6
13	14	15	16	17	18	19	
20	21	22	23	24	25	26	
27	28						

13
MONDAY

14
TUESDAY

15
WEDNESDAY

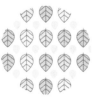

16
THURSDAY

17
FRIDAY

Last Quarter ☾ ## 18
SATURDAY

19
SUNDAY

February 2017

			1	2	3	4	5
6	7	8	9	10	11	12
13	14	15	16	17	18	19	week 7
20	21	22	23	24	25	26
27	28

20
MONDAY

21
TUESDAY

22
WEDNESDAY

23
THURSDAY

24
FRIDAY

25
SATURDAY

New Moon ◯ **26**
Solar Anular Eclipse SUNDAY

February 2017

		1	2	3	4	5
6	7	8	9	10	11	12
13	14	15	16	17	18	19
20	21	22	23	24	25	26
27	28					

week 8

Balasana

Child's Pose

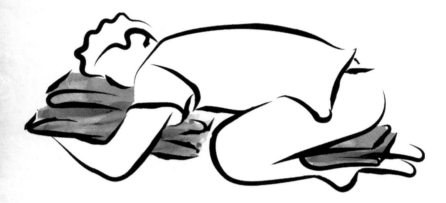

Coming into the Pose

- Kneel on the floor.
- Have one or more folded blankets in front of you.
- Sit back, bringing your heels towards your buttocks.
- Place another folded blanket between your heels and buttocks to cushion your knee joints.
- Separate your knees hip-distance apart (or as close or wide as you like).
- Exhale and fold forward, resting one cheek on the blankets.
- Allow your belly to rest between or on top of your thighs.
- Let your arms rest on the floor or gently hug the blankets.

While in the Pose

- Let go of your weight onto the blankets with each exhalation.
- Release your shoulders towards the ground.
- Breathe into your lower back.
- After some time, change cheeks to rest the other one on the blanket.

Coming out of the Pose

Place your hands on the floor, lengthen the front torso and gently lift up on an inhalation.

What the Prop Does for the Pose

The first blanket provides soft support and elevation to the chest and head. The second blanket cushions and creates space for the knee joints.

Benefits

- Stretches the lower back, ankles and knees.
- Calms the mind and body.
- Relieves fatigue.
- Can be used as resting asana anytime during a longer practice.

Contraindications

- Knee injury.
- Ankle injury.
- Diarrhoea.
- Advanced pregnancy.

Other Props for this Pose

Sandbag. A small sandbag placed on your lower back increases your sense of grounding. (See The Sequence, p.230)

Chair. Sitting on one chair and leaning forward onto the seat of another chair in front of you avoids compression on the knees.

For full instructions on these poses, check our blog *www.yogagendas.com/blog* each month during 2017.

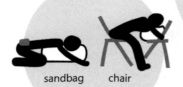

sandbag   chair

my notes

Keep Alkaline, Keep Healthy

By Elena Sepúlveda

As yogis, we know the importance of maintaining balance for wellbeing. Our diets, mind states, and environments are as much allies as challenges for keeping that crucial-for-health balance of acidity and alkalinity in our body tissues.

The human body regulates its many functions to achieve internal equilibrium through a biological process, called homeostasis, and this includes the vital regulation of acid-alkaline balance. An acidic body has been recognised as one of the major causes of diseases, such as early aging, cancer, diabetes, high blood pressure, osteoporosis, and many others. If its fluids turn too acidic, the body has alkaline reserves to neutralise them, but excess of acidity can deplete these reserves and weaken the immune system. This shift in body chemistry is called acidosis. We can consciously help the natural process of homeostasis through our food choices, yoga practices, and environmental habits.

An Alkaline Diet

Most organic fruits and veggies have an alkalinizing effect on the body and counteract acidity. The same can be said of delicious superfoods, like wheat, alfalfa, barley, oat, and kamut grass, and algae, like spirulina, chlorella, or kelp. At the other end of the spectrum, processed foods, meats, refined sugar, alcohol, coffee, and dairy products are highly acidifying. You will find many, good acid-alkaline food charts on the internet; a diet containing more foods from the alkaline side of the chart will always be healthier.

To help the alkalinising effects of a healthy diet, there is an Ayurvedic remedy said to eliminate toxins and excess acidity. Oil pulling has been used for centuries to clean gums, teeth, tongue, and other parts of the mouth.

It is simple, and it works best first thing in the morning after waking up. To do it, take a spoonful of organic cold-pressed sesame oil and swish it around in your mouth for a few minutes. Then spit it out, clean your tongue with a tongue scraper, and finally, rinse it with salty water.

An Alkaline Mind

According to Ayurveda, negative mind-sets can manifest in the body, creating imbalances, one of them being acidosis. The different pranayama techniques used in yoga help balance body chemistry, transforming negative mind-sets. When the breath slows down during pranayama, the parasympathetic nervous system is engaged, and this leads to a calmer state of mind.

The sympathetic nervous system is more active when stressed and breathing too quickly; then there is a build-up of oxygen in the bloodstream and a decrease in the carbon dioxide, which upsets the acid-alkaline balance of the blood. Breathing slowly, the levels of carbon dioxide rise again, and bodily functions can go back to homeostasis.

Yoga Chitta Vritti Nirodhah is sutra 1.2 in Patanjali's *Yoga Sutras*. It is translated as "yoga is the cessation of the fluctuations of the mind". Fostering focus and concentration through yoga, we are also cultivating a steady mind and helping the acid-alkaline balancing act in our bodies.

An Alkaline Environment

Environmental factors affect our acid-basic levels. Household cleaning products, commercial soaps, shampoos, cosmetics, etc. contain a chemical load that is very toxic to the body and contribute to acidosis. Many deodorants, for example, suppress sweating (a bodily function that helps to eliminate toxins) and push toxins back into the lymph nodes, weakening the immune system. When we purchase chemical-free products, we contribute to our own health and to that of the planet.

Essential oils are said to be highly alkalising. They are the plant essence and, therefore, have a frequency that the body and mind recognise. Like when we are in nature, breathing fresh air, essential oils can act as anti-oxidants, converting free radicals (associated with oxidative damage or stress, which causes chronic inflammation) into water and oxygen, especially citrus fruits and green plants essential oils. But, perhaps, the best alkaline environment is nature itself!

A Balancing Act

The body's pH needs to be in the middle, but slightly on the alkaline side of the scale. Standing for "potential for hydrogen", pH measures the hydrogen ions in body fluids, such as urine, blood, or saliva. Hydrogen ions dissolve acid, so the more hydrogen ions in a solution, the more acidic it is. The pH scale goes from 0 (most acid) to 14 (most alkaline).

The human body must have a pH of around 7.4 to function optimally. Remember this, like many things in life, is a balancing act.

my notes

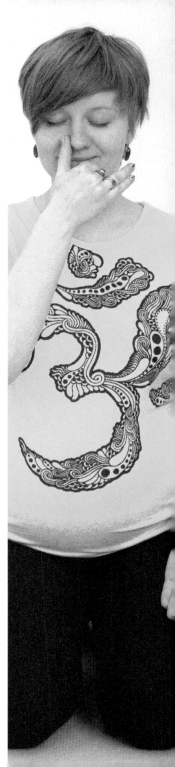

This month I will change

This month I will accept

This month I discovered

March 2017

March 2017

		1	2	3	4	5
6	7	8	9	10	11	12
13	14	15	16	17	18	19
20	21	22	23	24	25	26
27	28	29	30	31		

27
MONDAY

28
TUESDAY

1
WEDNESDAY

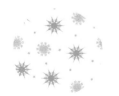

2
THURSDAY

3
FRIDAY

4
SATURDAY

First Quarter ☽ # 5
SUNDAY

	1	2	3	4	5	week 9
6	7	8	9	10	11	12
13	14	15	16	17	18	19
20	21	22	23	24	25	26
27	28	29	30	31		

6

MONDAY

7

TUESDAY

8

WEDNESDAY

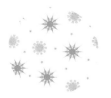

9
THURSDAY

10
FRIDAY

11
SATURDAY

Full Moon ○ **12**
SUNDAY

March 2017

		1	2	3	4	5
6	7	8	9	10	11	12
13	14	15	16	17	18	19
20	21	22	23	24	25	26
27	28	29	30	31		

week 10

13
MONDAY

14
TUESDAY

15
WEDNESDAY

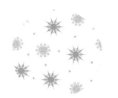

16
THURSDAY

17
FRIDAY

18
SATURDAY

19
SUNDAY

		1	2	3	4	5
6	7	8	9	10	11	12
13	14	15	16	17	18	19
20	21	22	23	24	25	26
27	28	29	30	31		

week 11

March 2017

20 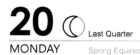 Last Quarter
MONDAY   Spring Equinox

21
TUESDAY

22
WEDNESDAY

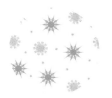

23
THURSDAY

24
FRIDAY

25
SATURDAY

26
SUNDAY

March 2017

		1	2	3	4	5
6	7	8	9	10	11	12
13	14	15	16	17	18	19
20	21	22	23	24	25	26
27	28	29	30	31		

week 12

PLANNER HANDBOOK JOURNAL | 75

27
MONDAY

28 ◯ New Moon
TUESDAY

29
WEDNESDAY

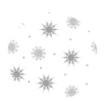

30
THURSDAY

31
FRIDAY

1
SATURDAY

2
SUNDAY

March 2017

		1	2	3	4	5
6	7	8	9	10	11	12
13	14	15	16	17	18	19
20	21	22	23	24	25	26
27	28	29	30	31		

week 13

Chaturanga Dandasana

Four Limbed Staff Pose or Plank Pose

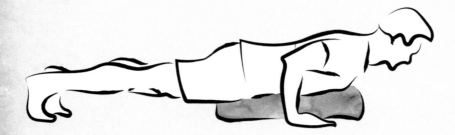

Coming into the Pose

- Place a bolster lengthwise in front of you.
- Lie face down on the bolster, keeping the top a few centimetres away from your collarbones.
- Let the prop support most of your body's weight.
- Point your toes on the floor and straighten your legs.
- Place the palm of your hands next to your lower ribs and keep your forearms as vertical as possible.
- Inhale and push with your hands on the floor with your elbows on top of your wrists.
- Keep your head in line with your spine.
- Engage your quadriceps and abdominal muscles.

While in the Pose

- Maintain your weight on the bolster without lifting your body off it.
- Squeeze your upper arms towards your ribs.
- Engage the front of your shoulders and chest and the back of your arms.
- As you press on the floor with your hands, engage your side body.

Coming out of the Pose

On an inhale, transition into Urdhva Mukha Svanasana (Upward Facing Dog), or bring your knees to the floor to exit the pose on an exhale.

What the Prop Does for the Pose

It does the heavy lifting so you can concentrate on aligning hands, arms and shoulders.

Benefits

- Strengthens the wrists and arms.
- Tones the abdomen.
- Strengthens the legs.
- Opens the chest gently

Contraindications

- Shoulder injury.
- Wrist injury.
- Carpal tunnel syndrome.
- Pregnancy.

Other Props for this Pose

Belt. Wrapping a belt around your upper arms stops you from lowering yourself too much and encourages proper alignment in the upper body.

Block. A block at different heights can be used to ease in and out of the pose while strengthening core and arm muscles.

For full instructions on these poses, check our blog *www.yogagendas.com/blog* each month during 2017.

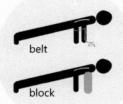

belt

block

my notes

Hatha Yoga: The Yang to Acupuncture's Yin

By Kayla Lakusta

In Traditional Chinese Medicine, one of the fundamental theories is that of Yin and Yang. The theory describes the way everything in the universe naturally pairs with opposites, and that these opposites are mutual complements. The same can be said for yoga: the word *Hatha* is literally translated as *Ha* (sun) and *Tha* (moon), a pair of mutually complementing opposites.

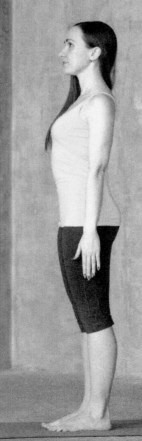

Bringing the body into one balanced state of yin and yang is the aim of both acupuncture and yoga.

One of the most important poses in yoga is Tadasana or Mountain Pose. If we look at this pose, we can start to see it and break it down ad infinitum into yin and yang aspects. The head reaching high to the heavens, and the utmost yang, in this case, is a mutual complement to the feet grounded down to the earth and utmost yin. Heaven and earth, head and feet, back and front, shoulders to fingertips, hips to toes, and on.

If we look at the most yang acupuncture point and highest point in the body, Baihui DU-20, we see its name is literally translated as One Hundred Meetings, referring to the convergence of all yang meridians in the body. When we are in Tadasana, we are reaching Baihui to the heavens.

If there is an excess of yang in the body, it can create a relative deficiency of yin in the body, and that person can feel ungrounded, hot headed, restless, and agitated, as the yin counterbalance has become too deficient to ground.

This can manifest itself in the yoga asana Tadasana. If the student lacks yin (grounding) and has an excess of yang (rising), it will be difficult to balance, holding still and strong. If we practice an inversion like Adho Mukha Vrksasana (Handstand), we can focus on grounding Baihui, bringing it to a more yin place, reducing the yang and strengthening the yin. Acupuncture can create the same balance by needling Yongquan KI1 at the bottom of the foot, highly effective for descending the energy in the body and grounding the yang.

We can also start to see how a person with excess yin would have difficulties holding a strong, firm Tadasana. An excess yin would create a relative deficiency in yang, and Bahui would lack strength to reach for the heavens getting full extension. This would also create issues if trying to hold Adho Mukha Vrksasana, as excess yin would try to keep close to the ground, low lying and heavy. In this case, Tadasana may be a great pose to practice by strengthening the yang, drawing up, lifting out of the heaviness of the yin with Baihui. In the case of a yin-excess individual, yang would be relatively deficient, so we could needle

Baihui to strengthen the yang and bring the counterparts back into balance.

If we look at these elements, we can see how all of them can mutually convert. We could take Tadasana into an inversion like Adho Mukha Vrksasana, and all aspects of Tadasana would convert to their complementary pair, with feet becoming yang and hands yin, hips yang relative to yin shoulders, shoulders yang relative to head, and so on.

Inquiring into one of the most fundamental, ubiquitous asanas of yoga like Tadasana, we see how connected everything in the universe is, using the theory of Yin and Yang.

Everything can be infinitely divided into yin and yang, and these opposite pairs depend on one another, counterbalance one another, and are mutually convertible.

We also see the balance of yin and yang is the true goal of both yoga and acupuncture and can be promoted with the practice of both yoga and acupuncture.

The asana limb of yoga is the yang to the yin of acupuncture treatment. Keep in mind, though, these are mutually transformable concepts, and that acupuncture can become the yang to yoga's yin. A mountain is only as high as the valley is low, so next time you're in Tadasana, check with your body: are you grounding your feet, rooting Yongquan, and extending your head reaching through Bahui?

Balance those opposites, and if one is feeling deficient, try strengthening it with an inversion or getting in for some acupuncture to help complement your practice on your mat.

Hatha:
Sun and Moon

A pair of mutually complementing opposites

my notes

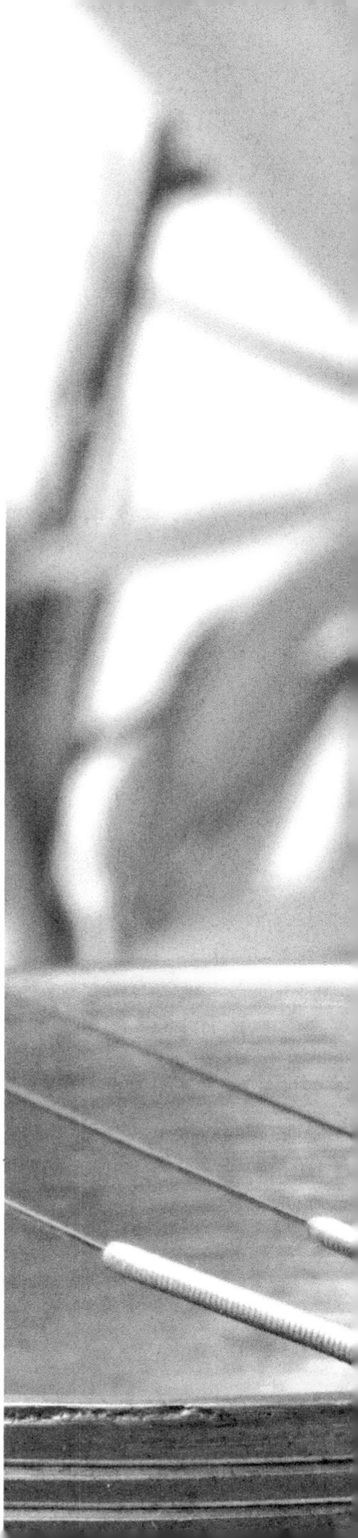

_____

_____

_____

_____

_____

_____

_____

_____

_____

_____

_____

_____

_____

_____

_____

_____

_____

_____

_____

_____

_____

_____

_____

_____

_____

This month I will change

This month I will accept

This month I discovered

April 2017

April 2017

					1	2
3	4	5	6	7	8	9
10	11	12	13	14	15	16
17	18	19	20	21	22	23
24	25	26	27	28	29	30

3 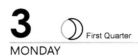 First Quarter

MONDAY

4

TUESDAY

5

WEDNESDAY

6
THURSDAY

7
FRIDAY

8
SATURDAY

9
SUNDAY

April 2017

					1	2
3	4	5	6	7	8	9
10	11	12	13	14	15	16
17	18	19	20	21	22	23
24	25	26	27	28	29	30

week 14

10
MONDAY

11 ○ Full Moon
TUESDAY

12
WEDNESDAY

13
THURSDAY

14
FRIDAY

15
SATURDAY

16
SUNDAY

					1	2
3	4	5	6	7	8	9
10	11	12	13	14	15	16
17	18	19	20	21	22	23
24	25	26	27	28	29	30

week 15

17
MONDAY

18
TUESDAY

19
◖ Last Quarter

WEDNESDAY

20
THURSDAY

21
FRIDAY

22
SATURDAY

23
SUNDAY

April 2017

					1	2
3	4	5	6	7	8	9
10	11	12	13	14	15	16
17	18	19	20	21	22	23
24	25	26	27	28	29	30

week 16

PLANNER HANDBOOK JOURNAL | 91

24
MONDAY

25
TUESDAY

26
 New Moon
WEDNESDAY

27
THURSDAY

28
FRIDAY

29
SATURDAY

30
SUNDAY

					1	2
3	4	5	6	7	8	9
10	11	12	13	14	15	16
17	18	19	20	21	22	23
24	25	26	27	28	29	30

week 17

Resting Bharadvajasana Twist

Bharadvaja's Pose

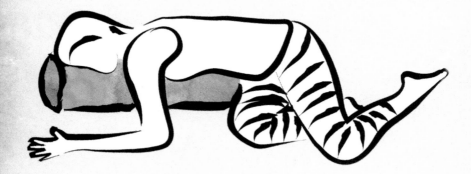

Coming into the Pose

- Sit in Dandasana (Staff Pose).
- Bend your legs back and place them beside your left hip.
- Place a bolster lengthwise on the floor and bring its end close to your right hip.
- Inhale and elongate your spine.
- On an exhale, turn your chest towards the bolster.
- Finish your exhalation by gently falling forward until your chest rests on the bolster.
- Allow your arms and hands to rest comfortably on the floor.
- Place your right cheek on the bolster.

While in the Pose

- Bring your knees towards the bolster as much or as little as feels appropriate.
- Make sure your feet are comfortably placed in relation to each other.
- Let go of your weight onto the bolster with each exhalation.
- Release your shoulders towards the ground.

Coming out of the Pose

Inhale and slowly push with your hands on the floor to lift up.
Remove the bolster and stretch out your legs. Repeat on the other side.

What the Prop Does for the Pose

It alleviates discomfort in the lower back and provides soft support
and elevation for the chest and head.

 ## Benefits

- Massages the abdominal organs and improves digestion.
- Alleviates lower back pain.
- Loosens stiff shoulders and neck.
- Helps relieve stress.

 ## Contraindications

- Knee injury.
- Advanced pregnancy.
- Lower back injury.
- Degenerative disk condition.

Other Props for this Pose

Cushion. If the forearms feel uncomfortable and don't reach the floor, you can place cushions under them for support. (See The Sequence, p.230)

Block. Raising the level of the bolster by putting a few blocks underneath alleviates lower back discomfort.
(See The Sequence, p.230)

For full instructions on these poses, check our blog *www.yogagendas.com/blog* each month during 2017.

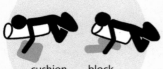

cushion   block

my notes

_____

_____

_____

_____

_____

_____

The Science of Movement and Music

By Derek Beres

Most comments after my yoga classes address the music. Since I began teaching in 2004, the playlist has been an integral component of the experience, equal in importance to the postures and transitions. With a background in dance, alongside being a world music journalist, the intersection of movement and music seemed a natural fit.

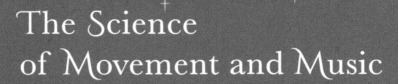

Music is the only evolutionarily unnecessary endeavor humans throughout time have all participated in. Food, shelter, and sex are required for our preservation.

Music hits our pleasure centers. It has been speculated that music predates language, acting as one of our species' first systems of communication. Regardless of origins, claiming music to be as necessary as breath is not an understatement.

Early in my own practice music was essentially an addendum in many classes I took around New York City. At the studio where I trained, there was no music. A stylistic choice: to use the elements and ambient sounds to lead you through the practice. Understandable, though not a style I could imagine teaching. I've come across practitioners who claim music is distracting to their practice. I remind them that's certainly one way to approach yoga. But it's not the only way.

Yet silence is preferable to the wrong music being played in a class. Of course, music is personal—we all have preferences, rang-ing from personal to social influences. Regardless of what we like, though, different music invokes differing chemical and physiological responses. Being armed with this information empowers movement professionals to make better choices when building their playlists.

I've been in classes in which the instructor played classical Indian music during aerobic sequences. According to a study conducted at the University of Berlin, sitar-based music lowers cortisol levels in the listener's blood.

While trying to increase our heart rates, the music was telling our brains to chillax. Conflicting messages between the movement and music did not create an optimal environment. I've also experienced instructors playing music with beats during Savasana. Also known as Corpse Pose, in honor of the deity Shiva's penchant for hanging around in cemeteries and smearing himself with ashes, Savasana is designed to physiologically relax the practitioner as much as possible. If a beat is playing, your heart rate increases, your lungs process oxygen more efficiently, and the area of your brain that controls movement is activated–things you'd never desire while trying to create a space for deep relaxation.

Tempo matters too: anything over 80 BPM (beats per minute) is probably going to activate the nervous system and motor neurons.

Lyrics activate the Wernicke's and Broca's areas of our brain–two regions that deal with the processing and application of language, adding another level of distraction.

Then there are minor keys, what we call 'sad music.' Oddly, the best time to listen to sad music is when we're... sad. Our brain treats listening to such music as positive. Research on why sad music feels pleasurable shows it to be a false loss, a fake psychic pain. Part of our brain has been fooled into thinking something terrible has happened, so we begin to empathize. Yet the more conscious cognitive part of our brain assesses the situation and reassures us that nothing bad has actually happened. The result is cathartic.

Music professor David Huron has linked this process to the hormone prolactin, which has a consoling effect: prolactin is released in mother's milk to calm a nursing baby. When people feel sad or begin to cry, prolactin is released throughout the body, and is measurable in blood and tears. Prolactin feels like a warm, fuzzy high. This is the brain taking care of us. Because nothing is wrong, our psychic release makes us feel consoled, a hormonal release without real tragedy occurring. Thus we feel good from this sad experience.

Knowing what music does to your brain and body only helps create a more powerful, more focused yoga experience–and focus is another thing music has been proven to aid.

It also ensures us that the brain/body divide that some schools have taught is an illusion. Consciousness is body-dependent: without all that wonderful chemistry orchestrated by our brain, metacognition (knowing that we know something) would be impossible.

If your yoga practice is about getting deeply inside yourself, sequencing the perfect soundtrack is a powerful and pleasurable means of doing just that.

my notes

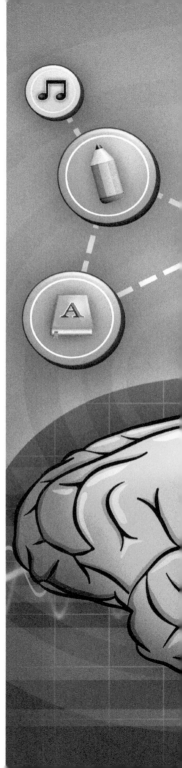

This month I will change

This month I will accept

This month I discovered

May 2017

May 2017

1	2	3	4	5	6	7
8	9	10	11	12	13	14
15	16	17	18	19	20	21
22	23	24	25	26	27	28
29	30	31				

1
MONDAY

2
TUESDAY

3
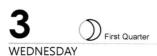 First Quarter
WEDNESDAY

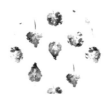

4
THURSDAY

5
FRIDAY

6
SATURDAY

7
SUNDAY

May 2017

1	2	3	4	5	6	7	week 18
8	9	10	11	12	13	14	
15	16	17	18	19	20	21	
22	23	24	25	26	27	28	
29	30	31					

8
MONDAY

9
TUESDAY

10
◯ Full Moon
WEDNESDAY

11
THURSDAY

12
FRIDAY

13
SATURDAY

14
SUNDAY

1	2	3	4	5	6	7
8	9	10	11	12	13	14
15	16	17	18	19	20	21
22	23	24	25	26	27	28
29	30	31				

week 19

15
MONDAY

16
TUESDAY

17
WEDNESDAY

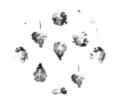

18
THURSDAY

Last Quarter ◖

19
FRIDAY

20
SATURDAY

21
SUNDAY

1	2	3	4	5	6	7
8	9	10	11	12	13	14
15	16	17	18	19	20	21
22	23	24	25	26	27	28
29	30	31				

week 20

22
MONDAY

23
TUESDAY

24
WEDNESDAY

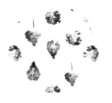

New Moon ◯ **25**
Super New Moon **THURSDAY**

26
FRIDAY

27
SATURDAY

28
SUNDAY

May 2017

1	2	3	4	5	6	7
8	9	10	11	12	13	14
15	16	17	18	19	20	21
22	23	24	25	26	27	28
29	30	31				

week 21

PLANNER HANDBOOK JOURNAL | 109

Parivrtta Parsvakonasana

Revolved Side Angle Pose

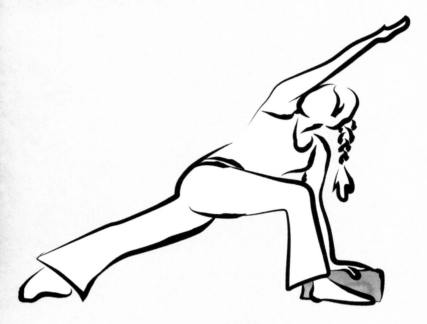

Coming into the Pose

- Stand in Tadasana (Mountain Pose), with a block near your feet.
- Inhale and step back with your left foot to approximately the distance of your leg's length.
- Keep your right foot looking forward at 90 degrees and turn your back heel in slightly. Align the right heel with the arch of the left foot.
- Inhale and grow tall.
- Exhale and bring both hips looking towards the front until you are facing over your right leg.
- On the next exhale, bend your right knee. On another exhale, turn further towards the right and lean the torso down, until you place your left hand on the block (bring it to the inner side of your right foot).
- Inhale and stretch your right arm over your head and over the back of your ear with the palm of the hand facing down.
- Turn your head to look towards your right hand.

While in the Pose

- Keep your back leg active extending through the back heel.
- Lengthen through your spine and the front of your body with each inhale.
- Rotate your chest open with each exhale, moving the diaphragm away from the abdomen.
- Soften your belly.

Coming out of the Pose

Inhale and come up. Turn to the front, straighten the knees and stretch the arms sideways. Exhale and step into Tadasana at the top of the mat, palms of the hands together in front of your heart. Repeat on the other side.

What the Prop Does for the Pose

It brings the floor closer to you if you can't reach it all that easily. It also aids balance.

Benefits

- Strengthens and stretches the legs, knees and ankles.
- Stretches the shoulders, back, chest, abdomen and hips.
- Improves balance.
- As with all twists, it stimulates the abdominal organs and improves digestion, in turn aiding elimination.

Contraindications

- Ankle, knee or neck injury.
- High or low blood pressure, insomnia or headaches.
- Pregnancy.
- Hernias.

Other Props for this Pose

Chair. Using a chair allows for maximal twisting motion (especially for people with larger bellies) and aids balance.

Cushion. The back knee can rest on a cushion and the twisting motion explored without the challenge posed by the balance.

For full instructions on these poses, check our blog *www.yogagendas.com/blog* each month during 2017.

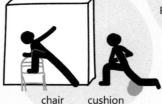

chair   cushion

my notes

Conscious Choices for Teacher Training

By David Lurey and Mirjam Wagner

Have you researched yoga teacher training programs on the Internet lately? You will discover the same challenges as when buying cereal in the supermarket: it is a daunting experience with dozens of choices! When shopping for cereal, you want something nutritious, ethical, and flavorful that fits your time and budget; yoga teacher training programs merit the same criteria research.

Nutrition

What do you want from your participation in a training? This is a great place to start. Intention is everything! Do you want to learn how to teach classes? To immerse yourself in asana practice? To meditate? To explore devotion and history? To develop body, mind, and spirit equally–or to develop one more than the others?

These are all addressed differently by teachers with varying degrees of priority. Make sure you will feel nourished by checking the curriculum, topics covered, and the teachers' focus. Talk to graduates, if possible, to find out as much information as you need about how and what is taught to be sure it fits your needs.

Ideally, you can/should meet the teachers in person, take at least one class or workshop from them, and make sure there is 'resonance.' Everything, including their voice, teaching style, philosophy, and way of life, will be transmitted in a training program, and these points should inspire you. If no direct contact is possible, first-hand recommendations from trusted sources are the next best thing. If possible, ask to talk to the teacher before investing your money and time with them.

The training location plays an important part in the nutritional value. Does it support your ability to focus and retreat from daily life to absorb as much as you can? Are you served healthy food? Does it encourage a conscious lifestyle? These are all personal preferences to investigate.

Ethics

Every human being in the world brings his/her own set of values to their lives. In a yoga training, the teachers are transmitting their values through words, thoughts, and actions. What ethical behaviors do you hold in your life that you wish to see in your teachers? Integrity? Authenticity? Discipline? Compassion? The ability to transmit knowledge and experience? Do you trust your teachers are able to lead you to yourself? Look closely before you commit to study with teachers, and be certain there is ethical alignment.

Flavor

Perfectly sweet with games and interactive lessons? Or 'just by the book'? Focus on alignment and poses? Perhaps with integrated philosophy? With mantras and meditation? There are so many flavors and approaches to teaching yoga that everyone's needs will be met! But will you find the course that fits your palate? Take some time to discover how you learn best and what teaching methods support you in learning and re-membering information, such as reading, listening, or doing.

Time and Budget

Training programs take many different formats, and this will play a big piece in your learning. Generally speaking, we can divide programs into two camps: immersions and periodic. Immersion-style courses, like we teach, are usually offered in a month-long residential style format. These courses have the potential to crack open deeper layers of personal development, as the time together with a group and the teachers digs deeper into the body-mind-spirit connection.

The challenge with these types of courses, often, is when you come home after being 'in the bubble' for several weeks with like-minded explorers, eating healthy food and making a commitment to personal growth in an environment that invites self-discovery.

Periodic courses are often better-suited for people who cannot take several weeks of their lives off. They spread their learning over several months or even years. These programs have the benefit of integrating yoga into daily life and putting concepts directly into action in the 'real world.'

However, with this broad ap-proach, the depth is often sac-rificed, as it is easier to fall back into old habits and patterns. Do you feel you are better served in a longer, more intensive program that digs to the core, but may be more difficult to put into daily life? Or are you better served spread-ing out the learning and integrat-ing it slowly, while needing other sources to uncover the deeper layers of habitual living?

These ideas can get you started on choosing the right training program and, hopefully, inspire and motivate you to listen to your intuition when choosing teachers... or cereal.

Nutrition Ethics
Flavor Time Budget

my notes

_____

_____

_____

_____

_____

_____

_____

_____

_____

_____

_____

_____

_____

_____

_____

_____

_____

_____

_____

_____

_____

_____

_____

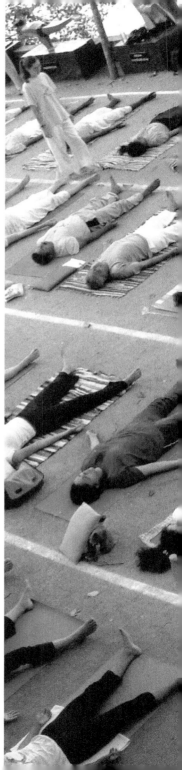

This month I will change

This month I will accept

This month I discovered

June 2017

June 2017

		1	2	3	4	
5	6	7	8	9	10	11
12	13	14	15	16	17	18
19	20	21	22	23	24	25
26	27	28	29	30		

29
MONDAY

30
TUESDAY

31
WEDNESDAY

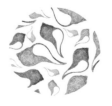

First Quarter 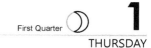 **1**
THURSDAY

2
FRIDAY

3
SATURDAY

4
SUNDAY

June 2O17

			1	2	3	4	week 22
5	6	7	8	9	10	11
12	13	14	15	16	17	18
19	20	21	22	23	24	25
26	27	28	29	30		

5
MONDAY

6
TUESDAY

7
WEDNESDAY

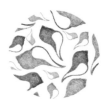

120 | YOGAGENDA 2017

8
THURSDAY

Full Moon ◯ **9**
Micro Full Moon **FRIDAY**

10
SATURDAY

11
SUNDAY

June 2017

				1	2	3	4
5	6	7	8	9	10	11		week 23
12	13	14	15	16	17	18
19	20	21	22	23	24	25
26	27	28	29	30

12
MONDAY

13
TUESDAY

14
WEDNESDAY

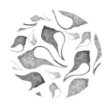

15
THURSDAY

16
FRIDAY

Last Quarter 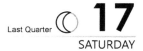 **17**
SATURDAY

18
SUNDAY

June 2017

			1	2	3	4
5	6	7	8	9	10	11
12	13	14	15	16	17	18
19	20	21	22	23	24	25
26	27	28	29	30		

week 24

19
MONDAY

20
TUESDAY

21
WEDNESDAY   Summer Solstice

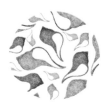

22
THURSDAY

23
FRIDAY

New Moon 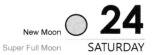 ## 24
Super Full Moon **SATURDAY**

25
SUNDAY

June 2017

			1	2	3	4
5	6	7	8	9	10	11
12	13	14	15	16	17	18
19	20	21	22	23	24	25
26	27	28	29	30		

week 25

26
MONDAY

27
TUESDAY

28
WEDNESDAY

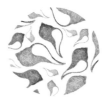

29
THURSDAY

30
FRIDAY

First Quarter ◐

1
SATURDAY

2
SUNDAY

June 2017

			1	2	3	4
5	6	7	8	9	10	11
12	13	14	15	16	17	18
19	20	21	22	23	24	25
26	27	28	29	30		

week 26

Upavistha Konasana

Wide Angle Seated Forward Bend

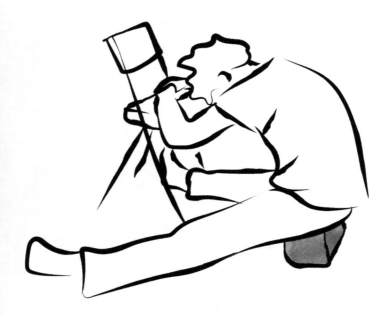

Coming into the Pose

- Sit on a block in front of a chair with its back away from you.
- Spread both legs apart.
- Inhale and elongate your spine.
- Exhale and hinge forward at the hip crease.
- Rest your arms on the seat of the chair.
- Rest your head on your forearms or on the seat of the chair if it is cushioned.
- Allow your spine to round naturally.
- Soften your legs as much as you need or even bend your knees slightly.

While in the Pose

- Allow your head to relax further onto your forearms or the seat of the chair on each exhale.
- Let your feet open to the sides if comfortable.
- Breathe towards the compression in the groin area.
- Feel the back of your neck stretching.

Coming out of the Pose

Inhale, slowly lift your head and move your body away from the chair. Move the chair to one side. Bring your legs together and bend your knees, hugging them to your chest.

What the Prop Does for the Pose

It elevates the hips and tilts the pelvis forward, softening the rounding on the lower back.

Benefits

- Stimulates the pelvic region.
- Stretches the inside and back of the legs.
- Releases the groin.
- Calms the mind.

Contraindications

- Lower back injury.
- Knee injury.
- Hamstring pull or tear.
- Groin pull or tear.

Other Props for this Pose

Weight. A weight placed on your lower back will add to your sense of grounding and awareness of this part of your body.

Bolster. Using a bolster instead of a chair allows you to go deeper into the forward bend while supporting your body and bringing the floor closer to you. (See The Sequence, p.230)

For full instructions on these poses, check our blog *www.yogagendas.com/blog* each month during 2017.

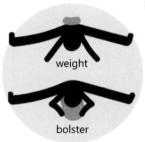

weight

bolster

my notes

Foot, Fascia, Spine: The Spring in our Step

By Gary Carter

Human postural control is a complex process of balancing the motions of all structures of the body in the field of gravity. Moving from one place to another would ideally be done by consuming a minimum amount of energy: bone, joints, ligaments, muscles and fascial tissues must be submitted to a minimum amount of stress. The very foundation of our moving structure can be considered to come from the foot and the spine.

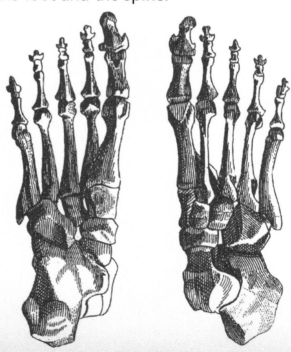

The foot is a structure that evolved to manage the surface below and the moving body above it. Disturbances here can have profound effects anywhere in our systems. With 26 bones, the foot mirrors the bones of the spine with the three basic arches that come into being during the first year of life. The bone shapes of the foot suggest its potential for efficiency, mobility, agility and strength; its multiple joints and tensioned fascial tissues and ligaments suggest it can manage the enormous loads and stresses put through it.

If the foot is a well-balanced structure with reasonably well organised and responsive arches, it can thrive on the forces and pressures.

The deeper surfaces of the foot have enormously strong, resilient ligamentous structures: plantar fascia, the deep plantar ligaments and the spring ligament.

These tissues comprise large amounts of collagen with a high tensile strength, meaning it has to be stiffer to take more load and return the energy of the load back up through the foot and leg. It can't be too elastic, as elastin deforms more quickly, swallowing some of the returnable energy. This returnable, usable energy is passed through the myofascial tissues and strong collagenous tissues of the leg.

Elasticities in the system can be considered not as quantities, but qualities that can be refined from the activity of the foot. For instance, the heel is a structure that can reach away from the base of the big toe in a subtle action repeated in postures, such as Tadasana (Mountain Pose), Adho Mukha Svanasana (Downward Facing Dog), Elbow Dog Pose, Utthita Chaturanga Dandasana (Plank Pose), helping to tension the tissues and the Achilles, returning energy back to the system to the deep fascial structure between the two bones of the lower leg, a tough collagenous membrane between the tibia and fibula, which accepts some of the returning energy. This potential ensures the muscles of the lower leg can be free to operate appropriately.

These forces can travel through the hamstring fascia and the deep adductor fascia, passing the energy to the spine, which utilises the energy from the foot and leg, harnessing a 'ground reaction force'.

Myofascial energy, deep stored fascial kinetic energy, can be released by the foot and leg. This process is harnessed, refined and trained through practice. Appropriate range through the foot, lower leg, adductors and hamstrings ensures no delay in communication.

The spine has the potential to use this energy to mobilise intervertebral joints, discs and tough spinal connective tissues. Discs pass the forces from one part to the next.

The pelvis and spine are wrapped in dense collagenous connective tissues, similar to the foot, storing and releasing enormous kinetic energy, allowing the varied and necessary undulations of flexion, extension, rotation and subtle side-bending motions. These are rhythmic in fashion, so the movements of walking and running can be as energy efficient as possible.

While standing, our proprioceptive system, which is our sense of where we balance ourselves in space, triggers immediate, precisely tailored and timed compensatory muscular contractions, reflexive in response to the changes, externally and internally.

We have an enormous amount of receptors in the plantar tissues in the foot; these feel heavy pressure, vibration, light pressure and skin stretch, and they divide into fast response and slow response. Widespread distribution of receptors throughout the plantar fascia shows the skin receptors constantly inform the nervous system and myofascial tissues of the terrain below and the movement above, responding in the most energy efficient way.

The thick connective tissue around the ankle, called retinacula, has a high percentage of proprioceptive nerve endings responsible for overall body balance. It is necessary to have free and balanced motion around the front of the ankle along with strong, mobile adaptive feet. Then returning energy from the foot can be passed through the system, utilised by the spine to allow for efficient movement.

Perhaps this can give potential for longevity to our tissues and help us maintain freedom of movement throughout our lives, which after all is our birth right!

my notes

This month I will change

This month I will accept

This month I discovered

July 2017

July 2017

					1	2
3	4	5	6	7	8	9
10	11	12	13	14	15	16
17	18	19	20	21	22	23
24	25	26	27	28	29	30
31						

3
MONDAY

4
TUESDAY

5
WEDNESDAY

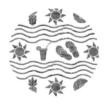

6
THURSDAY

7
FRIDAY

8
SATURDAY

Full Moon ◯ **9**
SUNDAY

July 2017

					1	2
3	4	5	6	7	8	9
10	11	12	13	14	15	16
17	18	19	20	21	22	23
24	25	26	27	28	29	30
31

week 27

10
MONDAY

11
TUESDAY

12
WEDNESDAY

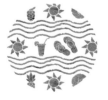

13
THURSDAY

14
FRIDAY

15
SATURDAY

Last Quarter ☾ 16
SUNDAY

July 2017

					1	2
3	4	5	6	7	8	9
10	11	12	13	14	15	16
17	18	19	20	21	22	23
24	25	26	27	28	29	30
31						

week 28

17
MONDAY

18
TUESDAY

19
WEDNESDAY

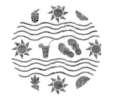

20
THURSDAY

21
FRIDAY

22
SATURDAY

New Moon ○ **23**
SUNDAY

July 2017

					1	2
3	4	5	6	7	8	9
10	11	12	13	14	15	16
17	18	19	20	21	22	23
24	25	26	27	28	29	30
31						

week 29

24
MONDAY

25
TUESDAY

26
WEDNESDAY

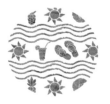

27
THURSDAY

28
FRIDAY

29
SATURDAY

First Quarter 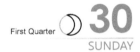 **30**
SUNDAY

July 2017

					1	2
3	4	5	6	7	8	9
10	11	12	13	14	15	16
17	18	19	20	21	22	23
24	25	26	27	28	29	30
31

week 30

Janushirsasana

Head to Knee Pose

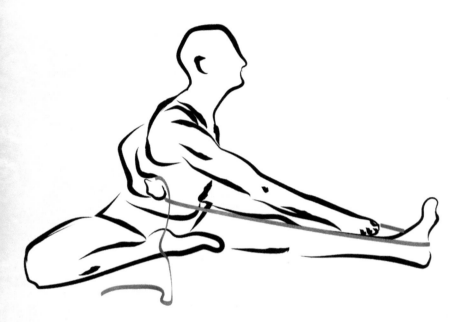

Coming into the Pose

- Sit in Dandasana (Staff Pose).
- Bend the right knee, bringing it towards your chest.
- Allow your right knee to fall open to the side. Make sure the sole of the right foot is touching the inner left thigh.
- Keep your left leg extended and your left foot flexed while pressing the top of your thigh down.
- Inhale and elongate your spine, exhale and twist very slightly to face the left leg.
- Loop a belt over the ball of the left foot and hold an end with each hand with your arms fully extended.
- On an exhale, hinge forward at the hip crease very slightly.
- After a couple of breaths, bring your left arm behind your back and get hold of the right end of the belt while holding the left end with the right hand.

While in the Pose

- Tuck the bottom of the left hip slightly back.
- Continue elongating your spine on the inhale while revolving the abdomen to the left.
- Continue bending gently from the hips on the exhale.
- Keep your back soft.

Coming out of the Pose

Inhale, come up and let go of the belt. Stretch the folded leg and feel your shoulders rest in line with your hips once again. Repeat on the other side.

What the Prop Does for the Pose

If the back rounds too much when reaching for the foot over the extended leg, the use of a belt allows you to explore the subtle motions of lengthening and bending from the hips without putting stress on the back.

Benefits

- Stretches the groins and hamstrings.
- Strengthens the back muscles.
- Elongates the front torso.
- Calms the mind and is said to relieve mild depression, anxiety and fatigue.

Contraindications

- Knee injury.
- Hamstring injury.
- Diarrhoea.
- Asthma.

Other Props for this Pose

Chair. Holding the seat of a chair while pushing with the foot of the extended leg against the lower bar of the chair helps the torso stretch and avoids collapsing the chest.

Blanket. Using a blanket under your buttocks allows the pelvis to tilt forward, making the pose more effortless.

For full instructions on these poses, check our blog *www.yogagendas.com/blog* each month during 2017.

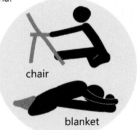

chair

blanket

my notes

Yoga for Autism

By David Ellams

Yoga4Autism is a UK-based center of excellence for bringing the wonderful and powerful magic of yoga to people with autism and cognitive disabilities, such as Down's syndrome and dyspraxia. In partnership with their training provider, Yo'Tism, they offer the most comprehensive method of neuro-sensory yoga in Europe tailored for special needs, especially autism.

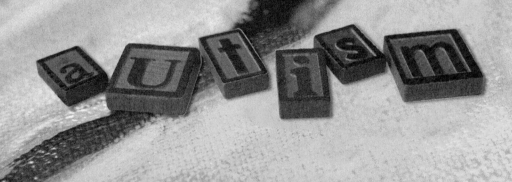

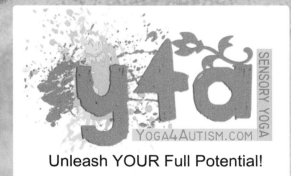

Unleash YOUR Full Potential!

At Yoga4Autism, we help people with special needs through the use of healthy natural methods such as yoga, mindfulness and meditation, nutrition and more to address the causes of their condition rather than covering up the symptoms with mind numbing drugs, as has been the way of the past. In doing so, we can help these people to live a happy and fulfilling life to their full potential and without limitations.

Sensory yoga, as taught by Yo'tism, offers a tool for equipping individuals with a diagnosis of autism and/or Asperger's syndrome as they regularly experience developmental or processing challenges, which often present themselves in a variety of symptoms requiring coping mechanisms.

Those on the spectrum need to work harder to 'be', as often, they are less connected to their bodies, more reactive to their environment, and their feedback systems can be greatly compromised.

95% of individuals on the spectrum have a sympathetic nervous system that is on 'red alert', and as a result, they have a limited bank of coping chemicals when faced with a perceived challenge.

Neuro-sensory yoga, a method based on using rhythmic movement and sound, helps keep individuals' 'internal tank' regulated throughout the day.

Sensory processing is how the brain processes information through the sensory receptors, and when this becomes distorted, input can seem threatening (hypersensitivities) or may not register at all (hypo-processing). Individuals on the spectrum experience this regularly, and incorporating yoga as part of a 'sensory diet' is a very powerful tool to bring the neuro-sensory system, body and mind into better balance, enabling the brain to filter information in a more integrated and clearer way.

Sensory yoga provides the sensory system the space to process, allowing the contracted muscles to relax slowly and bringing an individual a sense of internal control, which is calming and relaxing. The therapeutic body-brain integration of a neuro-sensory yoga sequence meets the needs, abilities and attention levels of an autistic individual and can take them from 'survival' mode to 'thriving' mode. This is achieved through incorporation of five different aspects of yoga: chanting, pranayama, asanas, relaxation and meditation, which enables channeling the flow of energy through the mind-body circuit, resulting in adjusting the chemical composition of the internal state and regulating the brain hemisphere imbalances.

Yoga4Autism offers a diverse range of yoga classes for children and adults. We also offer yoga for parents and carers so they can fully de-stress after a long day, before picking up their child or the person they are caring for. In addition to these, we run sessions for both children/adults and their parents/carers together, as this provides an excellent opportunity for them to bond and helps build vital social interaction skills. Our regular classes are taught in London and Brighton, but we can also come to you if there is demand, and help you get together with other parents/carers in your area.

A personal note

I'm David Ellams, the founder and director of Yoga4Autism, and I can personally vouch that our method works, since I myself am on the autism spectrum. I was given the label of Asperger's, dyspraxia and dyslexia, and after a lifetime of trying everything, with nothing working, I finally discovered yoga, mindfulness and meditation, which helped turned my life around in the most amazing way.

I have had a really hard life due to not having the help I needed. Now, I wish to help others so they do not have to suffer as I once did. I offer inspiring and empowering talks and a message of HOPE for people on the spectrum. As part of these talks, I detail various coping strategies I've developed over the years.

Further information about our work can be found on our website
http://www.yoga4autism.com

my notes

_____
_____
_____
_____
_____
_____
_____
_____
_____
_____
_____
_____
_____
_____
_____
_____
_____
_____
_____
_____
_____
_____
_____
_____
_____
_____
_____
_____
_____
_____

This month I will change

This month I will accept

This month I discovered

August 2017

August 2017

	1	2	3	4	5	6
7	8	9	10	11	12	13
14	15	16	17	18	19	20
21	22	23	24	25	26	27
28	29	30	31			

JOURNAL

31
MONDAY

1
TUESDAY

2
WEDNESDAY

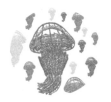

3
THURSDAY

4
FRIDAY

5
SATURDAY

6
SUNDAY

August 2017

1	2	3	4	5	6	week 31
7	8	9	10	11	12	13
14	15	16	17	18	19	20
21	22	23	24	25	26	27
28	29	30	31			

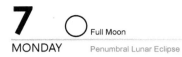

August 2017

7
MONDAY

○ Full Moon

Penumbral Lunar Eclipse

8
TUESDAY

Penumbral Lunar Eclipse

9
WEDNESDAY

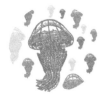

10
THURSDAY

11
FRIDAY

12
SATURDAY

13
SUNDAY

August 2017

	1	2	3	4	5	6
7	8	9	10	11	12	13
14	15	16	17	18	19	20
21	22	23	24	25	26	27
28	29	30	31			

week 32

14
MONDAY

15 ☽ Last Quarter
TUESDAY

16
WEDNESDAY

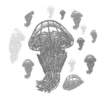

17
THURSDAY

18
FRIDAY

19
SATURDAY

20
SUNDAY

August 2017

	1	2	3	4	5	6
7	8	9	10	11	12	13
14	15	16	17	18	19	20
21	22	23	24	25	26	27
28	29	30	31			

week 33

21

New Moon

MONDAY

22

TUESDAY

23

WEDNESDAY

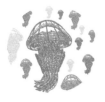

24
THURSDAY

25
FRIDAY

26
SATURDAY

27
SUNDAY

August 2017

	1	2	3	4	5	6
7	8	9	10	11	12	13
14	15	16	17	18	19	20
21	22	23	24	25	26	27
28	29	30	31			

week 34

28
MONDAY

29 ◗ First Quarter
TUESDAY

30
WEDNESDAY

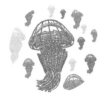

31
THURSDAY

1
FRIDAY

2
SATURDAY

3
SUNDAY

August 2017

	1	2	3	4	5	6
7	8	9	10	11	12	13
14	15	16	17	18	19	20
21	22	23	24	25	26	27
28	29	30	31			

week 35

Setubandha Sarvangasana

Supported Bridge Pose

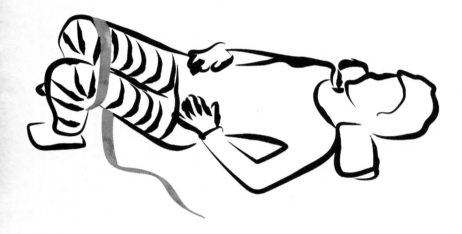

Coming into the Pose

- Place a carefully folded blanket on the floor.
- Exhale and lie on it on your back.
- Make sure your shoulders and head are off the blanket and on the floor.
- Put a rolled blanket under your neck.
- Bend your knees.
- Place your feet on the ground, approximately hip-distance apart and parallel.
- Wrap a belt around your thighs to hold your legs in place.
- Rest your hands on your abdomen.

While in the Pose

• Close your eyes and let the ground receive more of your weight on each exhale.

• Allow your legs to do a subtle internal rotation.

• Feel the soles of your feet rooted to the ground.

• Relax your shoulders, elbows and hands.

Coming out of the Pose

Unbind the belt and slowly hug your knees to your chest in Apanasana (Knees to Chest Pose). Roll onto your right side and sit up.

What the Prop Does for the Pose

It allows to let go and relax the legs completely while holding them in place.

Benefits

• Releases lower back tension.

• Rests the heart.

• Soothes the nervous system.

• Relieves ear and eye problems and headache.

Contraindications

• Sinus or respiratory issues.

• Back injury.

• Advanced pregnancy.

• This asana can be modified in different relevant ways and practiced by almost everybody.

Other Props for this Pose

Chair. Using a chair for support while back bending intensifies the chest opening effect of any asana of this type while liberating the legs and arms from the weight of the body. (See Viparita Dandasana, pp.178-179).

Block. A supporting block under the lower back can be used to open the front body and extend the back, while still keeping the pose passive and restorative.

For full instructions on these poses, check our blog *www.yogagendas.com/blog* each month during 2017.

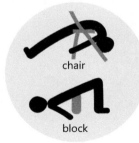

chair

block

my notes

Begin Again. And Again.

How Meditation Can Support Your Artistic Practice

By Karen Macklin

Even if you consider yourself a natural born artist, creative work can test your body, mind, and heart. Read on to find out how a daily meditation practice can help your creative efforts in very specific ways from a yogic perspective.

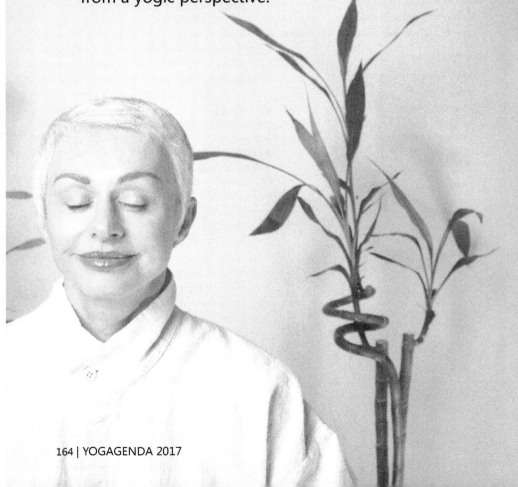

I'm a yoga teacher and a writer, but I was a writer first. I wrote my first poem at seven and my first play at nine. I started writing for magazines at 19, and went on to be a professional journalist, author, and playwright. I have written at times for money and at times for pleasure. I have written out of the desire to grow, the necessity to burn away layers of my past, and the impulse to let others to know they are not alone in this human heartland of tragedy, comedy, and mystery. Words are who I am, and how I am, and what I do.

But that doesn't mean that writing is easy. As any artist knows, creating is challenging–sometimes painfully so. It's hard on the body and it's hard on the mind and it's hard on the heart. It will keep you up at night, in the house on a beautiful day, and living just a little bit closer to the edge of your own soul. Meditation practice helps me stay committed, grounded, and open as an artist, and it offers a stronger sense of intention and meaning to my work.

From a yogic perspective, here's what artists have to gain from a daily meditation practice.

1. Meditation teaches us discipline (tapas).

One of the most challenging aspects of creative practice is carving out the time to do it. For most people, their creative discipline is not their primary form of income. This means that the rewards for creating are not external and immediate, but internal and long-term. If no one is lighting a fire underneath us to paint or make music, we have to light that fire ourselves. Daily meditation practice–even for five minutes–can teach us how to light that fire again and again. Slowly, the fire grows stronger, and is not extinguished so easily by mental distractions. We can then translate this skill of discipline to our artistic practice.

2. Meditation trains our concentration (dharana).

Distraction has likely been an impediment to artistic practice since our ancestors were pulled away from creating their cave-drawings to run from a wooly mammoth or engage in prehistoric primping. But today, distractions are no longer the interruption; they are the norm. More than ever, we need focus. Without it, we can sit down with our pens or pianos for hours and still get nothing accomplished. Simply training the mind to come back to the breath again and again is one of the best tools for strengthening our attention, which we can later direct to our art. When we practice deep concentration coupled with silence, we can also access states of emptiness, which are essential for the birth of new ideas.

3. Meditation teaches us the art of self-study (svadyaya), which enables us to attain states of clear-seeing (avidya).

Great art arises from a diversity of life experiences, and our ability to grow from them. In the same way we might travel to far flung corners of the globe to gain a deeper external experience of life, we can travel inward to gain a deeper internal experience of what it means to be human. The insights we gain from sitting quietly and reflectively with our own minds and bodies are invaluable doorways into the intricacies and complexities of our own subconscious. And because meditation shines a light on the clouded parts of our minds, it encourages us to see more clearly. Clear-seeing enables us to create not only from reactionary emotions like anger and fear, but from more refined emotions like compassion and love, which can make our art more empathic, intentional, and meaningful.

4. Meditation teaches us the practice of letting go (vairagya).

Some of the hardest challenges for artists happen not during the process of creating, but after the work is complete. We may believe that either our work or the response we receive after sharing it with others is lacking. Whether internal or external, rejection can break our hearts–plunging us into depression and possibly preventing us from continuing to create. Meditation teaches, with each breath, to let go of the last moment and move into the now. With patience and with practice, we learn to continually return to the present moment, where there is always the opportunity to start anew, to begin again.

Begin Again. And Again.

my notes

_____
_____
_____
_____
_____
_____
_____
_____
_____
_____
_____
_____
_____
_____
_____
_____
_____
_____
_____
_____
_____
_____
_____
_____
_____
_____

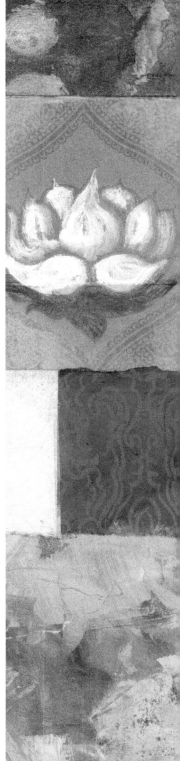

This month I will change

This month I will accept

This month I discovered

September 2017

September 2017

				1	2	3
4	5	6	7	8	9	10
11	12	13	14	15	16	17
18	19	20	21	22	23	24
25	26	27	28	29	30	

JOURNAL

PLANNER HANDBOOK JOURNAL | 169

4
MONDAY

5
TUESDAY

6
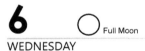 Full Moon
WEDNESDAY

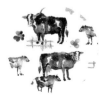

7
THURSDAY

8
FRIDAY

9
SATURDAY

10
SUNDAY

September 2017

			1	2	3
4	5	6	7	8	9	10
11	12	13	14	15	16	17
18	19	20	21	22	23	24
25	26	27	28	29	30

week 36

11
MONDAY

12
TUESDAY

13
Last Quarter
WEDNESDAY

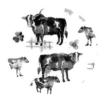

14
THURSDAY

15
FRIDAY

16
SATURDAY

17
SUNDAY

September 2017

				1	2	3
4	5	6	7	8	9	10
11	12	13	14	15	16	17
18	19	20	21	22	23	24
25	26	27	28	29	30	

week 37

18
MONDAY

19
TUESDAY

20
New Moon

WEDNESDAY

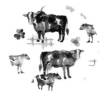

21
THURSDAY

22
Autumn Equinox   FRIDAY

23
SATURDAY

24
SUNDAY

			1	2	3	
4	5	6	7	8	9	10
11	12	13	14	15	16	17
18	19	20	21	22	23	24
25	26	27	28	29	30	

week 38

25
MONDAY

26
TUESDAY

27
WEDNESDAY

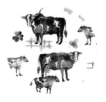

First Quarter ☽ **28**
THURSDAY

29
FRIDAY

30
SATURDAY

1
SUNDAY

				1	2	3
4	5	6	7	8	9	10
11	12	13	14	15	16	17
18	19	20	21	22	23	24
25	26	27	28	29	30	

week 39

Viparita Dandasana

Upward Facing Two Foot Staff Pose

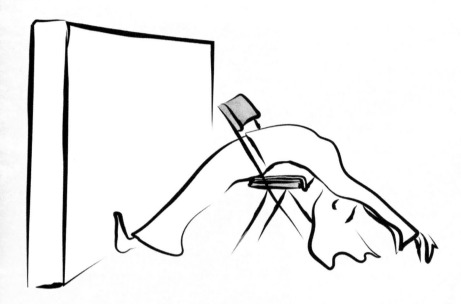

Coming into the Pose

- Place a stable chair away from a wall (at a distance approximately the length of your legs) with the back to it.
- Put a carefully folded blanket over its seat and front edge.
- Sit on the chair, taking your legs through the back and resting your sacrum on its back edge. Hold the back of the chair with both hands.
- Make your back concave and exhale, leaning back until your back ribs curve over the seat and your shoulder blades rest on the front edge.
- Place your toes against the wall and your heels on the floor, with your legs slightly bent.
- Take your arms under the seat and get hold of the back legs of the chair (or as close as you can reach).
- Straighten your legs, extend your trunk and allow your head to fall back.
- With your legs firm, take your arms over your head and stretch them towards the floor.

While in the Pose

- Stretch the back of your legs to firm them further.
- Allow your chest to open while your abdomen and ribcage stretch.
- Do not slide off the chair.
- Relax your head.

Coming out of the Pose

Inhale and look up. Slowly take your hands to the back of the chair again. Bend your legs and carefully come up, lifting your chest. Lean over the back of the chair for a few breaths to counter pose. Come out of the chair.

What the Prop Does for the Pose

It intensifies the chest-opening effect of this asana while liberating the legs and arms from the weight of the body.

Benefits

- Stretches the totality of the front body.
- Brings agility and longevity to the spine.
- Improves respiration.
- Invigorates the whole body.

Contraindications

- Spine nerve damage and disk problems.
- Cervical injury.
- High blood pressure and retinal problems.
- Pregnancy.

Other Props for this Pose

Bolster. A bolster placed crosswise on the mat under your middle and lower back allows for more ease and spaciousness to be created as your muscles can be totally relaxed.

Back Bender. Very similar to the deep chest opening provided by the chair, the back bender brings more stability to the pose.

For full instructions on these poses, check our blog *www.yogagendas.com/blog* each month during 2017.

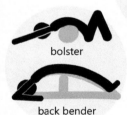

bolster

back bender

my notes

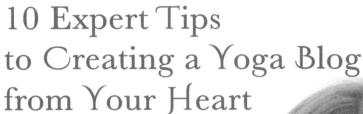

10 Expert Tips to Creating a Yoga Blog from Your Heart

By Michaela Olexova

If you feel the urge to express yourself, share and inspire others, blogging is the best creative platform to help you reach your tribe, wherever they are. Here are some useful suggestions from an expert blogger and yoga teacher.

I've never thought of blogging as something I should pick up just because it's trendy or I'm expected to. Writing and photography have always been my passion, since way before I wrote my first blog post, so for me, it was just a natural process to start a blog. There's so much I've learned over the years, so here is a small collection of tips I wish I had when I started out. Be creative, test them out and put them into action. And remember that at the end of the day, it's your life, your blog and your rules!

1. Getting started

It's important to be clear and decide what you expect your blog to do. Is blogging going to be your main thing, or is it just going to support and serve your primary yoga business? Clarity is the key as it helps you determine the choice and structure of your website as well as your work flow.

2. Finding your voice

Be real, honest and transparent and share from your heart! There's a chance that whatever inspires or excites you in this world may inspire thousands of other people. If you're not passionate about what you do, it will show in your blog posts and you'll lose your audience fast.

3. Authenticity

Don't be afraid to express yourself without fear of criticism. Blogging is about connecting and creating relationships, and there will always be people who love your work and resonate with you and those who don't. It's ok if they leave, because you wouldn't want to hang out with them anyway, right?

4. Consistency

If you want to take blogging seriously, you have to commit and create content consistently. It may take time, energy and money, so it's important to keep your focus and spirit high and hang in there. It will get easier as you learn what works and what doesn't. Ask for help if you get stuck; just get started and fine-tune things along the way.

5. Imagery

Don't underestimate the power of photos. There's nothing worse than pages of text with no images or very poor ones. It's the easiest way to grab peoples' attention and help them digest the information. Invest in a good camera or grab your iPhone and take advantage of free photo editing tools out there. Being creative and original can be as easy as pie!

6. Creating content

Start by listing things you're passionate about or you're the expert on, as they may hold a foundation to your blog structure, categories and tags. Demonstrations, interviews, how to guides, reviews, recipes, quotes, tips or behind the scenes are some favourites.

7. Inspiration

As you go out, talk to people, visit places and read or scan through Pinterest, you will be surprised how much inspiration is out there. Listen to conversations and ask your tribe about their passions, fears and desires. Can your blog posts help or support them in any way?

8. Style

To connect with your tribe, you have to be original! People don't want to see another version of someone else's blog, so don't copy or compare yourself to others. Why not start with a simple blog post with an enticing headline and a collection of beautiful images or a video? You develop your style as your confidence grows; just remember to use a language that sounds like you!

9. Scheduling

Try to create a blogging schedule in your calendar where you list all your posts at least 6 months in advance, you can always move around the dates and posts if you need to. If you can do 1-2 posts a month, that's great. If you can commit to a weekly post, you'll have more chances to get noticed.

10. Sharing

There are many ways to share your posts, and it's your job to let people know where they can find you. Set up a regular newsletter and find your fans in a few different places—from your social media platforms to guest blogging for an established blog or partnering with an inspiring brand.

The World is your Oyster!

my notes

This month I will change

This month I will accept

This month I discovered

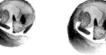

October 2017

October 2017

						1
2	3	4	5	6	7	8
9	10	11	12	13	14	15
16	17	18	19	20	21	22
23	24	25	26	27	28	29
30	31					

2
MONDAY

3
TUESDAY

4
WEDNESDAY

Full Moon ◯ **5**

THURSDAY

6

FRIDAY

7

SATURDAY

8

SUNDAY

October 2017

						1
2	3	4	5	6	7	8
9	10	11	12	13	14	15
16	17	18	19	20	21	22
23	24	25	26	27	28	29
30	31					

week 40

9
MONDAY

10
TUESDAY

11
WEDNESDAY

Last Quarter ☾ **12**
THURSDAY

13
FRIDAY

14
SATURDAY

15
SUNDAY

October 2017

						1
2	3	4	5	6	7	8
9	10	11	12	13	14	15
16	17	18	19	20	21	22
23	24	25	26	27	28	29
30	31					

week 41

16
MONDAY

17
TUESDAY

18
WEDNESDAY

New Moon ◯ **19**
THURSDAY

20
FRIDAY

21
SATURDAY

22
SUNDAY

						1
2	3	4	5	6	7	8
9	10	11	12	13	14	15
16	17	18	19	20	21	22
23	24	25	26	27	28	29
30	31					

week 42

23
MONDAY

24
TUESDAY

25
WEDNESDAY

26
THURSDAY

27
FRIDAY

First Quarter 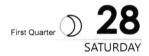 **28**
SATURDAY

29
SUNDAY

						1
2	3	4	5	6	7	8
9	10	11	12	13	14	15
16	17	18	19	20	21	22
23	24	25	26	27	28	29
30	31					

week 43

Viparita Karani

Legs Up the Wall Pose

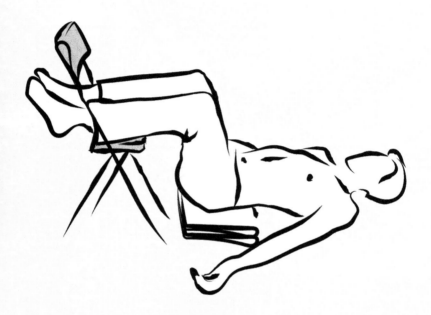

Coming into the Pose

- Place a few carefully folded blankets on the floor.
- Put a chair with its back away from you in front of the blankets.
- Sit sideways on the blankets.
- Slide 90 degrees around with the help of your hands and raise your legs to place them on the seat of the chair.
- Make sure your trunk has moved too and is in line with your legs.
- Exhale and lie back over the blankets, placing your head on the floor.
- Stretch your arms alongside your torso.
- Relax your hands, palms facing up.

While in the Pose

- Press your shoulders down.
- Allow the chair to take the whole weight of your legs.
- Become aware of the opening in the abdomen and chest.
- Relax your neck.

Coming out of the Pose

Remove one leg at a time from the chair and bring your knees towards your chest. Roll onto your right side and sit up.

What the Prop Does for the Pose

This pose is normally done with the legs up the wall (See The Sequence, p.230). If discomfort is felt with the legs extended along the wall, this variation with the chair provides relief while you still benefit from inverting the legs' blood flow.

Benefits

- Relieves lower back pain.
- Relaxes the legs and improves blood circulation.
- Allows blood to pool into the pelvis and abdominal region.
- Energises the body.

Contraindications

- Glaucoma.
- High blood pressure.
- Tightness in the hamstrings.
- Some traditions advice against this pose during menstruation.

Other Props for this Pose

Bolster. Lying on a bolster instead of blankets with legs up the wall provides support while intensifying the inverting effect. (See The Sequence, p.230)

Sandbag. A sandbag place on your feet in the legs up the wall variation of the pose grounds the sacrum and releases tension in the lower back.

For full instructions on these poses, check our blog *www.yogagendas.com/blog* each month during 2017.

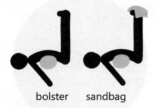

bolster   sandbag

my notes

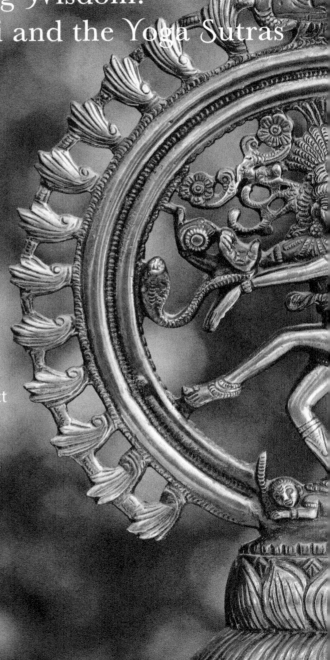

Renewing Wisdom: Patanjali and the Yoga Sutras

By Sattva Giacosa

Who was Patanjali? What are the *Yoga Sutras* about? There are rivers of literature and endless, enriching debates about these questions. There is also one fundamental aspect we can focus on understanding that will get us closer to our innate nature: bliss.

Once upon a time, thousands of years ago, or perhaps just now, in the realm of deities and extraordinary beings, the god Vishnu returned home in ecstasy after having witnessed the Ananda Tandava, the Dance of Joy. As he laid on his couch (the thousand headed serpent Adisesha), the snake looked at him and asked:

"Where are you coming from?"

"I'm coming from the forest, where I saw the Ananda Tandava!"

After listening to Vishnu's story, Adisesha asked, *"Could I too witness this dance?"*

And Vishnu replied, *"Of course, you can. But you must be born on Earth and search in the forest."*

Adisesha headed off for adventure. Meanwhile, in another realm of existence, there was a great yogini, named Gonika, sitting by the River Ganges, praying to the gods to be blessed with a son. Gonika was absorbed in her practice, her hands in Anjali Mudra (Prayer Gesture), when she suddenly felt something fall into her lap. As she opened her eyes, she saw a small being, half human and half serpent, who asked her to take him as a son. So she did, and she named him Patanjali.

Patanjali looked at her and asked, *"How can I witness the Dance of Joy?"*

Gonika replied, *"You have to follow your own nature as a snake and dig very deep into the earth until you can hear the drum of the Dance."*

That's how Patanjali dives into his own nature, searching for knowledge and navigating the depths until he hears the drum and finds the altar where the Dance of Joy is taking place.

We know little about Patanjali's life. There are no precise records of who he was, but there is a lot of debate about him. As with all mythological stories, this one can have endless interpretations. Personally, I believe one of the great teachings here is that we must always follow our innate nature and dig deep into who we are to be able to experience joy or bliss.

The first time I read *Light on the Yoga Sutras of Patanjali* by B.K.S Iyengar, I thought I'd never be able to learn even one sutra, nor understand them. And in some way, there is an element of truth in that, because the *Yoga Sutras* come from an oral tradition transmitted from teacher to student for thousands of years in a culture totally different than ours. The *Yoga Sutras* were not written initially; they were a means to pass on a whole body of philosophy in a concise and precise way, so it could be memorised and then conveyed when required. It was Patanjali who compiled them into a text.

Trying to understand Indian philosophical teachings from our rational and scientific viewpoint, believing that reading a book is gaining knowledge, is a big mistake. There is so much to understand in these teachings that the simple act of reading cannot let you comprehend the wisdom they hold. It is imperative to have a teacher to help us see how these philosophical concepts work on a day to day basis, instead of trying to apply them as dogmatic moral principles.

If we open a book on the *Yoga Sutras* and expand our knowledge of them, we need to understand they aren't linear teachings, and neither are the 8 Limbs of Yoga. It took me a long time to understand they were not a manual to be a yogi or yogini, but that they introduce us to the idea that we are enlightened from the beginning.

Samadhi Pada is the name of the first chapter in Patanjali's *Yoga Sutras*. If we look at this chapter closely, we see that Patanjali renders the idea that we already are in samadhi, or liberation, the same state of being we wish to reach through practice. It's around this concept that Patanjali compounds his teachings, offering us a method.

Patanjali is offering us tools and a concise method to get to know ourselves, not a means to conquer ourselves or fight against our human nature. More the opposite: he presents a thorough study of human nature's diversity and the different ways we can come closer to, observe, and accept that diversity, so we can find the path that best suits our human nature.

Our human nature: bliss

my notes

_____
_____
_____
_____
_____
_____
_____
_____
_____
_____
_____
_____
_____
_____
_____
_____
_____
_____
_____
_____
_____
_____
_____
_____
_____
_____
_____

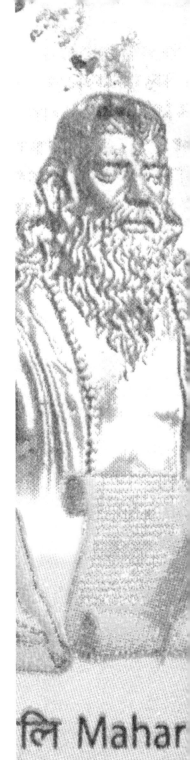

लि Mahar

This month I will change

This month I will accept

This month I discovered

November 2017

November 2017

		1	2	3	4	5
6	7	8	9	10	11	12
13	14	15	16	17	18	19
20	21	22	23	24	25	26
27	28	29	30			

30
MONDAY

31
TUESDAY

1
WEDNESDAY

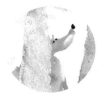

2
THURSDAY

3
Super Full Moon   ### FRIDAY

Full Moon 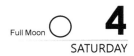 # 4
SATURDAY

5
SUNDAY

November 2017

		1	2	3	4	5
6	7	8	9	10	11	12
13	14	15	16	17	18	19
20	21	22	23	24	25	26
27	28	29	30			

week 44

6
MONDAY

7
TUESDAY

8
WEDNESDAY

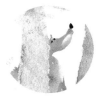

9
THURSDAY

Last Quarter ◖ # 10
FRIDAY

11
SATURDAY

12
SUNDAY

	1	2	3	4	5
6	7	8	9	10	11	12
13	14	15	16	17	18	19
20	21	22	23	24	25	26
27	28	29	30

week 45

13
MONDAY

14
TUESDAY

15
WEDNESDAY

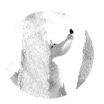

16
THURSDAY

17
FRIDAY

New Moon ⬤ **18**
SATURDAY

19
SUNDAY

November 2017

		1	2	3	4	5
6	7	8	9	10	11	12
13	14	15	16	17	18	19
20	21	22	23	24	25	26
27	28	29	30			

week 46

20

MONDAY

21

TUESDAY

22

WEDNESDAY

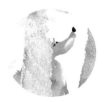

23
THURSDAY

24
FRIDAY

25
SATURDAY

First Quarter ☽ **26**
SUNDAY

		1	2	3	4	5
6	7	8	9	10	11	12
13	14	15	16	17	18	19
20	21	22	23	24	25	26
27	28	29	30			

week 47

27
MONDAY

28
TUESDAY

29
WEDNESDAY

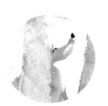

30
THURSDAY

1
FRIDAY

2
SATURDAY

Full Moon ○ ## 3
Super Full Moon SUNDAY

November 2017

	1	2	3	4	5	
6	7	8	9	10	11	12
13	14	15	16	17	18	19
20	21	22	23	24	25	26
27	28	29	30			

week 48

PLANNER HANDBOOK JOURNAL | 211

Sukhasana

Easy Pose

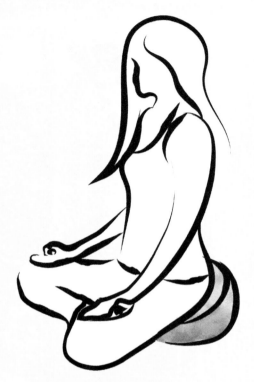

Coming into the Pose

- Sit on a cushion or zafu with your sitting bones near the front edge.
- Cross your legs and bring each foot roughly beneath the opposite knee.
- Allow your pelvis to tilt forward and your knees to reach or point towards the floor.
- Keep your back straight and soft.
- Place your hands beside each hip, cupping your fingers.
- Press with your fingertips on the ground while elongating your trunk towards the sky.
- Let your chin fall very slightly forward to create space at the back of your neck.
- Place your hands on your knees.

While in the Pose

- Close your eyes and breath evenly, deeply and consciously.
- Open your chest by bringing in the dorsal spine and widening the front ribs.
- Take your shoulder blades back and down.
- Relax your upper arms.

Coming out of the Pose

Open your eyes, move onto the next asana or close your practice by bringing your hands together in front of your heart for Namaste or a final mantra.

What the Prop Does for the Pose

It allows the pelvis to tilt forward, providing a steady base for the lower body while letting the hips gradually release and open.

Benefits

- Strengthens the spine.
- Opens the hips.
- Stretches knees and ankles.
- Calms the mind and supports meditation.

Contraindications

- Knee injury.
- Ankle injury.
- Hip injury.
- Weak back.

Other Props for this Pose

Block. Placing a block under each knee reduces the opening in the hips.

Blanket. Sitting on two or three folded blankets with knees level with the hips widens the knees and provide more hip space.

For full instructions on these poses, check our blog *www.yogagendas.com/blog* each month during 2017.

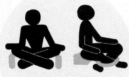

block   blanket

my notes

Yoga Teaching Stories

By Swami Saradananda

Everyone loves stories, including yogis.
What better way to understand yoga philosophy
than to hear a story that illustrates an esoteric
concept? The ancient rishis understood this
problem; they knew they were trying to convey
ideas that were often difficult to put into words,
so they made use of the transformative power
of teaching stories.

Each of the following classical teaching stories illustrates different aspects of yoga philosophy. As you read each story, allow it to enter your innermost being. Indian tradition holds there are basically three stages of connecting with stories:

• **Shravana:** you hear or read it.

• **Manana**: you think about it and analyse it using your intellect.

• **Dhyana:** you meditate on it, nourish it with your practice and let it purify and strengthen your resolve. Then, when properly assimilated, you feel the essence of the story taking the form of living inspiration.

The Blind People and the Elephant

Four blind people received special permission from a zoo to 'see' an elephant. The first person touched the leg and reported that an elephant is like a tree trunk. The second touched the side of the elephant and 'saw' that an elephant is like a brick wall. The third touched the trunk and knew from his own direct personal experience that an elephant was like a large snake. The fourth touched the tail and 'understood' that an elephant is similar to a piece of rope. Then they all started fighting because each believed that she/he knew the true nature of the elephant.

In relation to the Infinite, we are all like these blind people. We each have a different relationship and viewpoint, and thus we 'see' things differently. Each person has a different understanding of the world because her/his point of view is different. None of us can really understand the Infinite— because we are each using our finite minds.

When you begin your yoga practice, your perception of the Infinite is imperfect. With regular meditation and constant self-analysis, you begin to experience the interconnectedness and completeness of all life.

The Snake in the Rope

One night a man was walking home alone in an area where there were no streetlights. In the dark, he stepped on something that seemed like a snake—and it bit him. He fell down, clutching his leg and shouting for help.

His neighbour came out with a lantern to see what was the matter. When the man told him that he'd been bitten, the neighbour asked where the snake was—best to know if it was a poisonous one or not. The 'bitten' man pointed to a bush, and when the neighbour shone his lantern on it, they realised that it was actually a piece of rope that appeared snakelike in the dark.

Just as the man superimposed the idea of a snake onto the piece of rope, our minds superimpose this world onto the infinite Reality.

The rope remains a rope, whether we believe it to be a snake or not. The rope doesn't change when our understanding changes. Similarly, the reality of the world does not change, but our understanding of it can be illumined by the light of knowledge.

The Farmer and the Donkey

One day a donkey fell into a well and started to cry pitifully. His owner tried, but couldn't figure out how to get him out. Finally the farmer came to the conclusion that as the donkey was old and the well needed to be covered up anyway, it wasn't worth the effort to retrieve the donkey. Instead, he began shovelling dirt into the well to fill it up.

At first the donkey cried even more horribly. Then, he quieted down. Looking into the well, the farmer was amazed at what he saw.

As each shovel of dirt hit the donkey's back, he would shake it off and step up onto it. As the shovelling continued, he stepped higher and higher. Soon the donkey stepped over the edge of the well and trotted off.

Life is going to shovel all sorts of dirt onto you. The trick is to shake it off and use it as a lesson to step up. That way each failure becomes a stepping-stone towards success. You can overcome the deepest problems by never giving up! Shake it off and use the apparent failure as a lesson to take a step up!

my notes

This month I will change

This month I will accept

This month I discovered

December 2017

December 2017

				1	2	3
4	5	6	7	8	9	10
11	12	13	14	15	16	17
18	19	20	21	22	23	24
25	26	27	28	29	30	31

December 2017

4
MONDAY

5
TUESDAY

6
WEDNESDAY

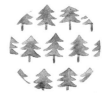

7
THURSDAY

8
FRIDAY

9
SATURDAY

Last Quarter ☾ # 10
SUNDAY

December 2017

			1	2	3
4	5	6	7	8	9	10
11	12	13	14	15	16	17
18	19	20	21	22	23	24
25	26	27	28	29	30	31

week 49

December 2017

11
MONDAY

12
TUESDAY

13
WEDNESDAY

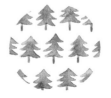

14
THURSDAY

15
FRIDAY

16
SATURDAY

17
SUNDAY

December 2017

				1	2	3
4	5	6	7	8	9	10
11	12	13	14	15	16	17
18	19	20	21	22	23	24
25	26	27	28	29	30	31

week 50

December 2017

18
MONDAY

New Moon

Micro New Moon

19
TUESDAY

20
WEDNESDAY

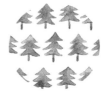

21
Winter Solstice   THURSDAY

22
FRIDAY

23
SATURDAY

24
SUNDAY

December 2017

				1	2	3
4	5	6	7	8	9	10
11	12	13	14	15	16	17
18	19	20	21	22	23	24
25	26	27	28	29	30	31

week 51

December 2017

25
MONDAY

26 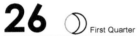 First Quarter
TUESDAY

27
WEDNESDAY

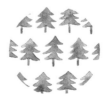

28
THURSDAY

29
FRIDAY

30
SATURDAY

31
SUNDAY

December 2017

			1	2	3
4	5	6	7	8	9	10
11	12	13	14	15	16	17
18	19	20	21	22	23	24
25	26	27	28	29	30	31

week 52

Savasana

Corpse Pose

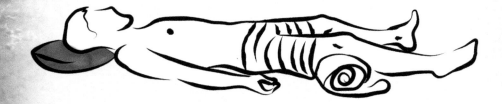

Coming into the Pose

- Sit in Dandasana (Staff Pose).
- Exhale and lean back onto your elbows.
- Further lower your back to the ground vertebra by vertebra.
- Place a rolled blanket under your knees and relax your legs.
- Place a cushion under your head to slightly bring your chin towards your chest.
- Extend your arms alongside your body, palms of the hands facing up.
- Allow your ankles to relax and your feet to drop out.
- Close your eyes.

While in the Pose

- Relax your facial muscles, paying special attention to your jaw and forehead.
- Let your body sink into the ground.
- Quieten your breathing.
- Invite your mind to remain calm and present.

Coming out of the Pose

Become aware of your toes and fingers and start moving them slowly.
Wake your body up little by little and make any gentle movements you feel like doing.
Roll onto your right side. Sit up in Sukhasana (Easy Pose) to close your practice.

What the Prop Does for the Pose

A cushion placed under the head brings the chin towards the chest,
creating space in the cervical vertebrae at the back of the neck.

Benefits

- Calms the central nervous system, and therefore the mind.
- Lowers high blood pressure.
- Alleviates stress and mild depression.
- Helps with insomnia.

Contraindications

- Sinus or respiratory issues.
- Back injury.
- Advanced pregnancy.
- This asana can be modified in different relevant ways and practiced by almost everybody.

Other Props for this Pose

Blanket. A blanket under the body cushions your back and increases your sense of being supported by the earth.

Eye Pillow. It blocks the external light, relieving tension and calming the active muscles around your eyes.

For full instructions on these poses, check our blog *www.yogagendas.com/blog* each month during 2017.

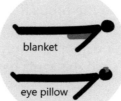

blanket

eye pillow

The Sequence: Restorative Yoga to Ease Anxiety

by Carol Trevor

This sequence of six poses focuses on creating calm and ease through the experience of rooting and connecting to the earth. It provides stability and containment for the body, while gently encouraging a comfortable amount of opening in areas that can feel constrained, i.e., the chest, back and abdomen. The limbs and head are supported, leading to soothing quiet for the mind.
No effort is required and the body is left to feel blissfully comfortable.

You can cover yourself with a blanket in all these poses to feel further care and wellbeing. Allow the hands to gently hold the props if needed. Keep your eyes open if you prefer, with the gaze lowered. Stay in the poses for a shorter amount of time and gradually build up if this feels better for you.

Enter and exit each pose slowly and mindfully. Pause for a few breaths between each pose. Be open to experiencing any sensations that arise in the practice without needing to question or analyse them.

Photos © Franco Satalino, 2016. francosatalino@gmail.com

Points of focus:

1. Feel the support of the props and the ground.

2. Feel the weight of your body. Where does it feel heaviest? Surrender the weight of your body to the props and ground.

3. Feel the breath. Focus on your exhalations, as this leads to a calm and peaceful mind. If the mind is busy, focus on equalising the length of the inhalations and exhalations, for example by counting to three for each breath. Once that is comfortable, lengthen the exhalations by one or two counts. If the mind is not busy, stay with natural, uncontrolled diaphragmatic breathing throughout.

1. Balasana (Child's Pose)

Place the knees on either side of the end of the bolster and fold forwards. Begin with one cheek on the bolster and change to the other side half-way through. Palms can be on the ground or loosely around the bolster.

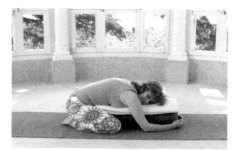

Modifications:
if you feel tightness in the hips or lower back, increase the height of the bolster by placing blankets on top of it. A blanket under the knees, ankles and between the heels and buttocks is also helpful to cushion and create space for the joints. To exit, place the palms on the floor and gently push yourself up to sitting.

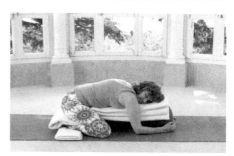

Holding time: 4 minutes

2. Resting Bharadvajasana (Bharadvaja's Pose) Twist

Sit on your heels with your right hip at the thin end of your bolster. Allow your feet to come out to the left side. The left foot rests above the right, with as much space between the knees and lower legs as you need. Inhale and raise your right arm. As you exhale, turn your chest towards the bolster and fold forwards onto it as your palms reach the floor. Your head can turn to the left or to the right if comfortable. Let your arms rest on the floor or gently hold the bolster. Place a blanket under the head if comfortable. To exit, bring your head to centre and press your palms into the ground to gently lift up. Repeat on the other side.

Modifications:
to accommodate any tightness or discomfort in the lower back, hips or hamstrings, raise the level of the bolster with blocks or cushions. Place cushions under the forearms if they don't easily reach the floor. Place a blanket between the knees.

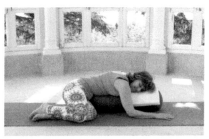

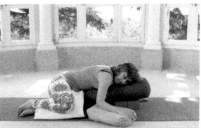

Holding time: 1-2 minutes each side

3. Upavistha Konasana (Supported Wide Angle Pose)

Sit on one or two blocks or cushions to elevate the hips. Exhale and slowly lean forward, resting the forearms on the ground and the head on a bolster and as many cushions as you need. Ensure the legs remain in line, without rolling forward. The knees are soft.

Modifications:
lean forward onto a chair and place a rolled-up blanket under the knees. The knees can bend if needed. Rest the head on the forearms and cushions. The spine can round naturally.

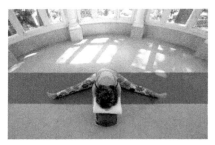

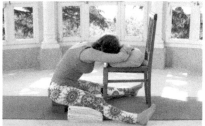

Holding time: 3 minutes

4. Setubandha Sarvangasana (Supported Bridge Pose)

Lie on a folded blanket with the shoulders and head on the mat. The feet are against a wall and gently bound with a belt. Place a blanket or weight on the abdomen for grounding and breath awareness. Place an eye pillow on the forehead to reduce sensory stimulation. Palms can be up or down or rested on the abdomen. To exit, bend the knees towards the chest and roll over to one side to sitting.

Modifications:
if there is any discomfort in the lower back, bend the knees and place the feet parallel on the blanket. Gently bind the thighs with a belt, so the legs remain restful.

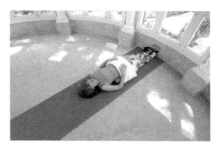

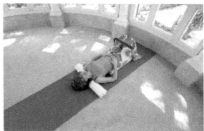

Holding time: 5 minutes

5. Viparita Karani (Legs Up the Wall Pose)

Create a gentle elevation by lying on a folded blanket with your seat against the wall. To enter, sit sideways to the wall, lean back, turn and allow the legs to come up naturally against the wall. Place a blanket or weight on the abdomen, an eye pillow on the forehead and a rolled blanket or towel under the neck. Allow the arms to rest naturally at the sides of the torso or place the hands on the abdomen. To exit, bend the knees towards the chest and roll over to one side to sitting.

Modifications:
if you experience pins and needles in the legs or feel tightness in the hamstrings, bend the knees and place the lower legs on a chair.

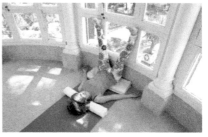

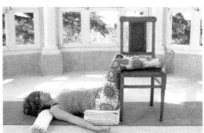

Note: this pose is not suitable during menstruation. Holding time: 3 minutes

6. Savasana (Corpse Pose)
Chest Elevated / Side Version

Elevate the chest slightly by placing a folded blanket under the middle and upper back. Elevate the head and place a rolled towel or blanket under the neck. The chin should point downwards slightly.
Place an eye pillow on the forehead or a crepe bandage around the head if this is comfortable for you.

Modifications:
lie on your left side. Place cushions between the knees, a bolster behind your back and a cushion in front of your chest to gently hug. Place the head on cushions.

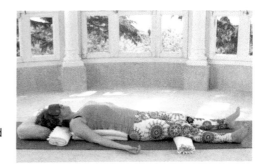

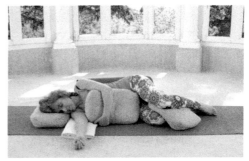

Holding time: 5-10 minutes

To seal the practice, slowly come to a comfortable seated position. Sit for a few moments. Notice how you feel. Journal your experiences if you wish.

All props kindly provided by **YogaYe.com** / Your Yoga Online Store

Asana Index

Yoga Events and Meditation Centres around the Globe

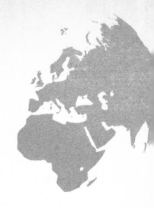

Curated by Michelle Taffe from
theglobalyogi.com

For up to date information on these events and more check
www.theglobalyogi.com/events/category/festivals-conferences

JANUARY

Meditation Centre of the Month:

Gaia House, UK

A meditation retreat centre in Devon, England that offers silent meditation retreats in the Buddhist tradition. Hosted in a stunning Manor House, dating to the 16th century, Gaia House is a sanctuary of contemplative calm, set amongst the gentle hills and quiet woodlands of South Devon.

www.gaiahouse.co.uk

Evolve Yoga and Wellness Festival

(Various Locations, Australia)

1 day for the coming together of the Southern Hemisphere yoga and wellness community in Byron Bay, Melbourne and Sydney.

www.evolveyogafestival.com.au

Kundalini Yoga Festival

(San Esteban, Chile)

7 days of Kundalini yoga practice, expanding on the teachings of Yogi Bhajan in the mighty Chilean Andes.

www.festivalkundalini.com

FEBRUARY

Meditation Centre of the Month:

Spirit Rock, USA

Dedicated to the teachings of the Buddha as presented in the Vipassana tradition. In woodsy Marin County, Spirit Rock is a thriving community of mindfulness practitioners, offering a full schedule of retreats, teachings and talks. Spirit Rock also welcomes volunteers in many roles and time periods.

www.spiritrock.org

Austria Yoga Conference

(Wels, Austria)

3 days of yoga and music. A relative newcomer to the yoga conference circuit, the Austria Yoga Conference brings yogis and musicians together in this small Central European nation.

www.yoga-conference.at

Texas Yoga Conference

(Texas, USA)

3 days of yoga, motivational speakers and fun musical evening concerts in Houston.

www.texasyogaconference.com

Canon Beach Yoga Festival

(Oregon, USA)

3 days of yoga, art, health, wellness treatments, spa and fun on the Pacific Northwest coast of the US.

www.cannonbeachyogafestival.com

MARCH

Meditation Centre of the Month:

Moulin de Chaves, France

Housed in a stunning late 19th century chateau in the Dordogne in southern France, this is a meditation centre that teaches Vipassana in the Thai forest tradition. They offer retreats from May to September in meditation as well as yoga and related practices. The Moulin also welcomes short-term and longer-term volunteers.

www.moulindechaves.org

International Yoga Festival

(Rishikesh, India)

7 days on the banks of the sacred river Ganga; a week long celebration of yoga and one of the world's largest yoga events.

www.internationalyogafestival.com

Yogafest

(Dubai, UAE)

3 days of yoga in a tranquil outdoor setting in Dubai. This is a free, sustainable community event supported by volunteers and sponsorships.

www.yogafest.me

Spirit Fest

(Cape Town, South Africa)

3 days in the crisp mountain air practising yoga, meditation, mantra chanting and more with the core mission of creating community around mindful living in Cape Town.

www.spiritfest.co.za

Bali Spirit Festival

(Bali, Indonesia)

5 days of yoga and spiritual workshops, fabulous concerts given by well-known international musicians, healing and community, all magnified by the magical spirit of the island of Bali.

www.balispiritfestival.com

APRIL

Meditation Centre of the Month:

Wat Kow Tham, Thailand

Located on the beautiful and peaceful tropical island of Koh Phagnan in Thailand, this is an active Buddhist monastery hosting a community of monks. The Wat offers 7-day Vipassana meditation retreats that start on the 10th of each month for interested visitors. There is also the possibility to stay longer.

www.kowtahm.com

Yoga and Holistic Europe Meeting

(Merano, Italy)

2 days over a weekend completely dedicated to finding harmony through yoga practice in the South Tyrol.

www.yogameeting.org

Byron Spirit Festival

(Byron Bay, Australia)

3 days of inspirational yoga, music, tantra and dance in beautiful Mullumbimby, Byron Shire.

www.spiritfestival.com.au

Yoga Journal Conference: New York

(New York, USA)

5 days of yoga with classes in all styles and for all levels.

www.yjevents.com/ny/

MAY

Meditation Centre of the Month:

The Buddhist Retreat Centre, South Africa

Just 90 minutes from Durban, it offers a tranquil environment for the study and practise of philosophy, psychology, meditation, yoga and Buddhist arts. Organised retreats are offered throughout the year. The centre looks out across a vista of valleys, forests and rolling hills in the blue distance.

www.brcixopo.co.za/

Shakti Fest

(Joshua Tree, USA)

3 days to celebrate the devotional path through dance, yoga, kirtan, and meditation in California.

www.bhaktifest.com

Yoga Festival

(Padua, Italy)

2 days for yoga with teachers from around the world investigating new trends, ancient traditions and meeting new friends in Northern Italy.

http://www.yogafestival.it

Midsummer Festival of Yoga

(Dorset, England)

4 days of 'celebrating diversity in yoga' with workshops, discussions, music, dance and more in the English countryside.

www.yogafestival.org.uk

German Yoga Conference

(Cologne, Germany)

4 days to 'find freedom' in Cologne, at one of the most established yoga gatherings in Europe.

www.yogaconference.de

JUNE

Meditation Centre of the Month:

The Holy Isle, Scotland

Holy Isle is a small island on the west of Scotland with an ancient spiritual heritage dating to the 6th century. The founder and visionary for this project is Lama Yeshe Rinpoche, a Tibetan Buddhist meditation master in the Kagyu tradition. From April to October, the island's centre hosts guests for personal and group retreats.

www.holyisland.org

Colourfest

(Dorset, England)

4 days of celebrating life through the 'colours' of yoga, music and dance. A wonderful space in which to meet, play, connect and inspire.

www.colourfest.co.uk

The Great British Kundalini Yoga Festival

(Berkshire, England)

5 days of yoga in a friendly, nurturing environment of joy, devotion and service to all beings, rooted in the Kundalini yoga teachings of Yogi Bhajan.

www.kundaliniyogafestival.org.uk

Hanuman Festival

(Boulder, USA)

4 days of community-orientated, world-class yoga and mind-blowing music set at the foot of Colorado's Rocky Mountains.

www.hanumanfestival.com

Bhakti Yoga Summer

(Chiemsee, Germany)

3 days of love, yoga and music in the Bavarian countryside. Join in celebrating the 'flowering of the heart'.

www.bhaktiyogasummer.com

Solstice Yoga Festival

(Latvia)

3 days celebrating the European summer solstice near Riga. Yoga, flowers, special foods and singing to celebrate the season in this thousand year old Latvian tradition.

www.solsticeyogafestival.com

Dutch Yoga Festival

(Terschelling, The Netherlands)

3 days immersed in yoga on a Dutch island, enjoying beaches, camping, lake swimming, cycling and more.

www.yogafestival.info

Bhakti Fest Midwest

(Madison, USA)

3 days celebrating devotion through music, chanting, yoga, meditation and community in Wisconsin.

www.bhaktifest.com

JULY

Meditation Centre of the Month:

Shambala Mountain Centre, Colorado

Set in a mountainous valley in the Colorado Rockies, this is a place for retreat and introspection in the Buddhist tradition. Founded over 40 years ago by Chögyam Trungpa Rinpoche, it offers year-long programs in yoga and meditation, creative arts, relationship, family and work, retreat and renewal, and many more subjects.

www.shambhalamountain.org

Wanderlust Festival

(Aspen and the Squaw Valley, USA)

4 days to share yoga in rural Colorado or California together with great yoga teachers, musicians, artists and performers.

www.wanderlustfestival.com

Berlin Yoga Festival

(Berlin, Germany)

4 days to cherish 'every breath you take' in yoga, outdoors at the Kladow Kultural Park.

www.yogafestival.de

Bliss Beat Festival

(Sezzadio, Italy)

4 days in the Italian countryside sharing the magic of yoga and devotional kirtan.

www.blissbeatfestival.com

Barcelona Yoga Conference

(Barcelona, Spain)

5 days of inspiration in Barcelona with a team of renowned and dedicated teachers offering their personal vision of the ancient yogic wisdom.

www.barcelonayogaconference.cat

Telluride Yoga Festival Midwest

(Telluride, USA)

4 days of yoga, hiking, social events, music, meditations, SUP yoga, Ayurvedic dinners, all-day workshops and more in this picturesque valley hidden in the mountains of Colorado.

www.tellurideyogafestival.com

Ängsbacka Yoga Festival

(Molkom, Sweden)

7 days in the Nordic countryside focusing on Ahimsa: bringing peace and freedom to yourself and the world, with yoga enthusiasts of all levels and traditions.

en.angsbacka.se

AUGUST

Meditation Centre of the Month:

Wat Buddha Dhamma, Australia

A Buddhist monastery set in the lush mountainous country north of Sydney, Australia. Forming part of the lineage of the great Thai monk Ajahn Chah, the Wat is home to a small community of monks and lay people who welcome visitors for formal retreats or personal retreats of varying duration.

www.wbd.org.au

European Yoga Festival

(Fondjouan, France)

9 days of Kundalini yoga following the teachings of Yogi Bhajan, in a fairytale-like French chateau in a forest. Swim in one of two lakes on the property in between yoga sessions!

www.3ho-kundalini-yoga.eu

Finger Lakes Yoga Festival

(Ithaca, USA)

4 days to celebrate yoga, music and art in the stunning countryside of Ithaca, New York State. This is a rustic, community-orientated festival.

www.fingerlakesyogafestival.org

Wake Up Festival

(Colorado, USA)

5 days to 'wake up' in the mountains of Colorado. This festival is designed to engage, inspire, connect and awaken body and soul through talks, ritual and celebration.

www.wakeupfestival.com

SEPTEMBER

Meditation Centre of the Month:

Passaddhi Meditation Centre, Ireland

A small meditation centre seeking to make the teachings of the Buddha and, in particular, the meditation practices of Vipassana and Metta (loving-kindness) available to as many people as possible. It runs meditation retreats during the summer months led by various teachers from around the world and sometimes welcomes volunteers.

www.passaddhi.com

Bhakti Fest

(Joshua Tree, USA)

4 days celebrating devotion through music, chanting, yoga, meditation and community in California.

www.bhaktifest.com

Yoga Festival

(Rome, Italy)

3 days over a weekend completely dedicated to finding harmony through yoga practice in Rome.

www.yogafestival.it

Geneva Yoga and Music Festival

(Geneva, Switzerland)

5 days of yoga, kirtan, acrobatics, massage and more with a focus on creating peace in the heart of a multicultural community.

www.genevayogamusicfestival.ch

OCTOBER

Meditation Centre of the Month:

Lama Tzong Khapa Institute, Italy

Located in Tuscany and founded in 1977, the Institute has grown into one of the largest centres for Tibetan Buddhism in Europe. It houses a permanent Sangha of monks and nuns, an international body of lay students and visitors, and it welcomes everyone interested in following one of their courses or retreats or just spending time in a beautiful, peaceful setting.

www.iltk.org

Kundalini Yoga Asia Festival

(Thailand)

5 days dedicated to serve, inspire and empower humanity to be healthy, happy and whole through the teachings of Kundalini yoga.

www.kundaliniyogaasia.org

NOVEMBER

Meditation Centre of the Month:

The Abbey, Oxford, UK

A centre for spiritual retreat in a stunning medieval hermitage, once home to Benedictine monks in the 13th century. Just 10 miles south of Oxford, it has a year-round community that cultivates a spiritual life, while caring for the centre's buildings and exquisite garden. It offers silent meditation retreats throughout the year and welcomes volunteers.

www.theabbey.uk.com/

Yoga Festival

(Milan, Italy)

3 days over a weekend completely dedicated to finding harmony through yoga practice.

www.yogafestival.it

Namaste Festival

(Jakarta, Indonesia)

3 days bringing yoga, healing and related disciplines to Jakarta with the goal of making the Indonesian capital an international wel-lbeing destination.

www.namastefestival.com

DECEMBER

Meditation Centre of the Month:

Casa Werma (Shambala Centre), Mexico

Located in the central Mexican state of Michoacan, this is a practice and retreat centre for special programs, personal retreat, contemplation, art, and discovery. A part of the international Shambala network of meditation centres around the world, founded by Chögyam Trungpa Rinpoche, it offers a full program of retreats year-round.

www.casawerma.shambhala.org

Uplift Festival

(Byron Bay, Australia)

3 days to listen to global pioneers from all walks of life come together to share their gifts. Discover the limitless possibilities that emerge when we unify our visions for the greater good of all.

www.upliftfestival.com

Who Contributed to Yogagenda 2017

One more year I'm thrilled and honoured to have all the wonderful teachers, whose biographical notes appear below, contributing to Yogagenda. I have to confess that commissioning content is almost my favourite part in the creation of this publication. Sometimes I'm nicely surprised by an email from a teacher offering a fascinating and fitting contribution. Other times I approach a person whose work I admire and respect. As an editor, a yoga teacher and a yoga student, their contributions help me reflect on my own practice, my own teaching and the direction they are heading.

In charge of the 'visual side of it all' this year's edition is lucky to count again on a wonderful illustrator who has been with us from the beginning, a new creative graphic designer and talented photographer (biographical notes below too).

I trust all contributors' work is an inspiration to you throughout the year, in whichever way it's beneficial to your unique human experience. I also hope their insights, expertise, and 'personal flavour' enrich your practice and your life, fuel your curiosity, and expand your understanding and enjoyment of this fantastic resource called yoga.

Elena

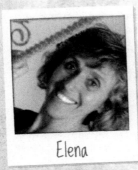

Elena

Elena Sepúlveda

(Keep Alkaline, Keep Healthy; Asana Overview; Asana Pages)

As founder, publisher, and editor of *Yogagenda*, Elena is the beating heart of this project that brings together her love for yoga and her passion for publishing. She is a yoga teacher (Vinyasa and Yin) and a body worker (Chavutti Thirumal), as well as a freelance writer and translator. Her aim is to blend both facets creatively and to find enjoyable and beneficial ways to share the results.

www.seed-joy.com

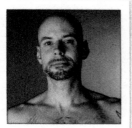

Derek

Derek Beres

(The Science of Movement and Music)

Derek is a Los Angeles-based author, music producer, and yoga/fitness instructor. He has taught at Equinox Fitness since 2004, developing a national yoga, music, and neuroscience program. He is a columnist for BigThink.com and 24 Life, 24 Hour Fitness's magazine and is the co-founder of EarthRise SoundSystem.

www.derekberes.com

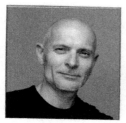

Gary

Gary Carter

(Foot, Fascia, Spine: The Spring in our Step)

Gary has been teaching yoga and PT for 30 years. Trained in the Scaravelli tradition, he has a keen feeling for the nature of fascia and movement and has worked with Thomas Myers in Structural Integration and the *Anatomy Trains* theory. Gary teaches Anatomy and Movement to yoga, pilates, and massage schools in the UK and Europe, and runs yoga TTCs from his own centre, Natural Bodies.

www.naturalbodies.co.uk

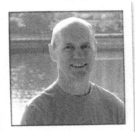

Bernie

Bernie Clark

(The Yinside of New Year's Resolutions)

Bernie is a meditation and yoga teacher, creator of the www.YinYoga.com website, and author of several books on yoga from the Western scientific viewpoint and the Eastern traditional viewpoints. His ongoing studies have taken him deeply inside mythology, comparative religions, psychology, physiology and anatomy. These explorations have clarified his understanding of Eastern practices and their value to Westerners.

www.yinyoga.com

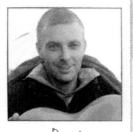

David

David Ellams

(Yoga for Autism)

David is founder & Managing Director of Yoga4Autism.org. Diagnosed with dyspraxia, dyslexia and Asperger's, he has managed to turn his life around with yoga and mindfulness. He has a First Class Honours Degree in Computing & Informatics and is rated one of the top IT contractors in the UK. He has used his successful career to get Y4A and NextGen Software off the ground.

www.yoga4autism.org

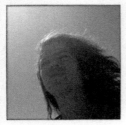

Sattva

Sattva Giacosa

(Renewing Wisdom: Patanjali and the Yoga Sutras)

Sattva has been a Barcelona-based yoga teacher for the last 10 years. In Vedic philosophy, sattva refers to purity in an enlightened sense. It is also her given name, a gift from her yoga practitioner parents. Spiritual and grounded, she teaches a non-dogmatic style with an emphasis on proper alignment and relaxed flow, with plenty of explanations and personalised attention.

www.sattvayoga.es

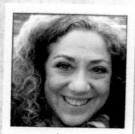

Lisa

Lisa Kaley-Isley

(Yoga for Seasonal Sadness)

Lisa is an experienced Para yoga teacher initiated into the Sri Vidya lineage and empowered to impart mantra and meditation practices. She is also a PhD Clinical Psychologist and Viniyoga trained yoga therapist enabled to design personalized prescriptive practices for individuals struggling with anxiety, depression, eating disorders, and the effects of trauma.

www.theyogitree.co.uk/lisa-kaley-isley

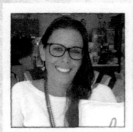

Kayla

Kayla Lakusta

(Hatha Yoga: the Yang to Acupuncture's Yin)

Kayla is a graduate of Alberta College of Acupuncture and TCM, and a member of the Alberta Governing Board of Acupuncturists. Kayla's passion for Eastern philosophy drives her in life. Making connections with like-minded people and sparking ideas fuel Kayla to be an active participant and a creative and involved practitioner.

www.banyantreehealth.com

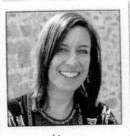

Karo

Karoline Leopold

(Graphic Design for *Yogagenda* 2017)

Karo is a German graphic designer and illustrator based in Barcelona. She worked in the design and publicity team of a big company before she started turning her passion for drawing into a profession by earning a Master's Degree in children's book illustration in Cambridge, UK. Back in sunny Barcelona, she works as a freelancer. She loves dancing and travelling whenever possible!

www.karolineleopold.com

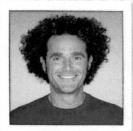

David

David Lurey

(Conscious Choices for Teacher Training)

Radiating enthusiasm and love, David Lurey teaches Vinyasa yoga for a connection to the self; Acroyoga for connecting to other humans; Green yoga as a way to connect more deeply with the planet and cosmos and Bhakti yoga for divine connections. It is his passion to create intelligent and inspiring yoga classes and workshops that touch body, mind and spirit at every chance.

www.findbalance.net

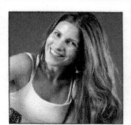

Karen

Karen Macklin

(Begin Again. And Again. How Meditation Can Support your Artistic Practice)

Karen is a writer and yoga teacher. Her articles have appeared in a myriad of publications, including Yoga Journal, Tricycle, and the New York Times. Her plays have been staged in NYC, SF, and beyond. She is an experienced yoga teacher (500-ERYT), who lives and teaches in San Francisco and leads local and international retreats.

www.karenmacklin.com

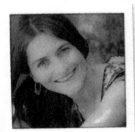

Michaela

Michaela Olexova

(10 Expert Tips to Creating a Yoga Blog from Your Heart)

Michaela is a Prana yoga teacher, website designer and business mentor for well-being professionals and heart-centred businesses, and founder of Business of OM. She's also a mama to a beautiful daughter, soul seeker, traveller and a great believer that you can have the life and business of your dreams... if you really want to.

www.michaelaolexova.com

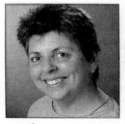

Saradananda

Swami Saradananda

(Yoga Teaching Stories)

Swami Saradananda is an internationally renowned yoga-meditation teacher who inspires you to want to practice. She is the author of a number of books, including *Chakra Meditation, The Power of Breath, Essential Guide to Chakras* and *Mudras for Modern Life*. After working with Sivananda Yoga Centres for many years, she undertook intensive personal practice in the Himalayas. Now based in London, she teaches workshops and courses worldwide.

www.flyingmountainyoga.org

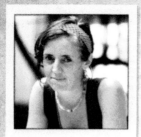

Michelle

Michelle Taffe

(Yoga Events and Meditation Centres around the Globe)

Michelle is a yogi, writer, musician, traveller, digital maven and the founder of The Global Yogi, a web platform that connects yogis with retreat centres and yoga and spiritual events worldwide. Michelle is also half the team from the e-course YourFabYogaLife.com, which helps people build a thriving professional life in yoga and wellness. Michelle is based in Australia and travels regularly, reporting on yoga and the spiritual path worldwide.

www.theglobalyogi.com

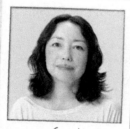

Carol

Carol Trevor

(Introduction to Restorative Yoga;
The Sequence: Restorative Yoga to Ease Anxiety)

With over 25 years' experience of yoga, Carol has a passion for sharing its quiet practices: pranayama, Restorative, yoga Nidra and meditation as a means of enjoying peace, vibrant health and fulfilment in everyday life. She is a dedicated practitioner, teacher and teacher trainer based in the UK, and the creator of a series of progressive yoga Nidra downloads.

www.yogacarol.co.uk

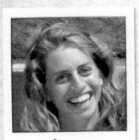

Denise

Denise Ullmann

(Yogagenda's logo; Illustrations for Asana Pages)

Denise was born in Buenos Aires. She is an osteopath and practises Acroyoga and contact dancing. She has painted for as long as she can remember. Since she began studying arts, she has worked on a variety of projects, such as illustrating logos for festivals, postcards, and stories related to art and meditation. She has also edited her own first illustrated book, *Asai Va*, and loves to paint big pictures.

www.abriendounmundo.blogspot.com

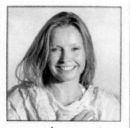

Mirjam

Mirjam Wagner

(Conscious Choices for Teacher Training)

Mirjam focuses on transmitting the wisdom of the human body and its close connection to emotional experiences in a simple, transparent, and very effective way. Sarah Powers is her most significant influence for Buddhism, mindful awareness and daily meditation practice.

www.yogatherapymallorca.com

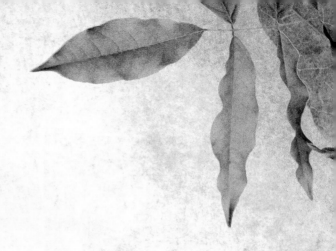

Sanskrit Glossary

Ananda Tandava: the Dance of Joy; a divine dance performed by the god Shiva, the source of the cycle of creation, preservation and dissolution.

Anjali Mudra: hands joined together in front of the heart; a gesture practiced throughout Asia and beyond and used as a sign of respect, greeting or when praying.

Asana: pose or posture; third stage in Patanjali's eight-limbed path of yoga.

Avidya: false understanding, ignorance, confusion.

Bhagavad Gita: a sacred text, part of the Indian epic Mahabharata, where the god Krishna teaches yoga to his devotee Arjuna.

Dharana: concentration; sixth stage in Patanjali's eight-limbed path of yoga.

Dhyana: meditation; seventh stage in Patanjali's eight-limbed path of yoga.

Hatha: sun and moon; union of the opposites.

Kirtan: group chanting, usually as a call-and-response.

Kriya: practice aimed at cleansing the body.

Manana: the stage of reflection on the teachings; thinking about and analysing them with one's intellect.

Mantra: sacred sound.

Marga: path.

Namaste: a spoken greeting or salutation commonly used in India. Often translated as "May the good in me honours the good in you".

Niyama: five self-observances relating to the inner world; second stage in Patanjali's eight-limbed path of yoga.

Pranayama: breathing technique; fourth stage in Patanjali's eight-limbed path of yoga.

Pratyahara: sensory withdrawal; fifth stage in Patanjali's eight-limbed path of yoga.

Purusha: pure consciousness, one's true self regarded as eternal and unaffected by external circumstances.

Raja yoga: the path of meditation; one of the four main margas or yoga paths mentioned in the Bhagavad Gita as ways to reach Liberation.

Rishi: seer, sage, wise elder.

Samadhi Pada: first chapter in Patanjali's *Yoga Sutras*. It defines yoga and the stages of consciousness.

Samadhi: ecstasy or pure awareness; the eighth and last stage in Patanjali's eight-limbed path of yoga.

Sattva: one of the three gunas or essential qualities characterised by purity, light and vital balance.

Shravana: hearing or reading the teachings.

Sutra: lit. thread; aphorism about the yogic lifestyle by the sage Patanjali.

Svadyaya: the study of yoga texts; one of the five niyamas in Patanjali's eight-limbed path of yoga.

Tapas: discipline; one of the five niyamas in Patanjali's eight-limbed path of yoga.

Trataka: candle gazing; one of six cleansing techniques or kriyas.

Vairagya: dispassion or detachment.

JOURNAL

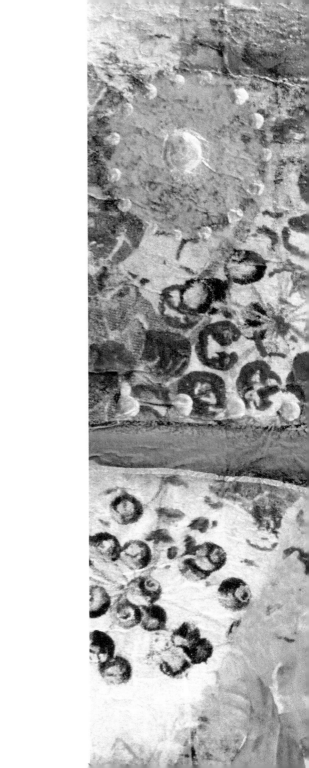

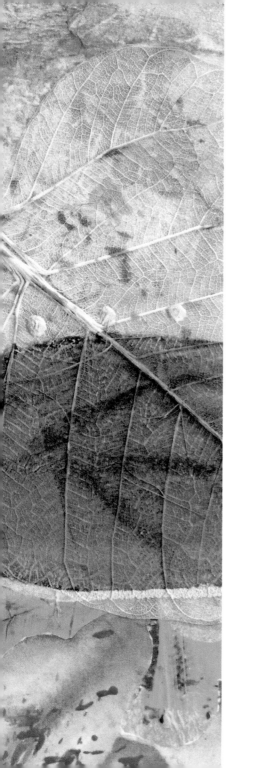

JOURNAL

JOURNAL

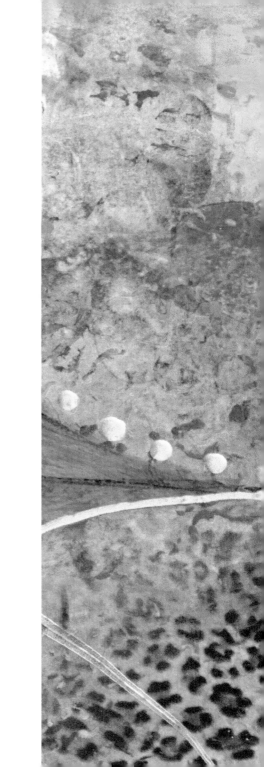

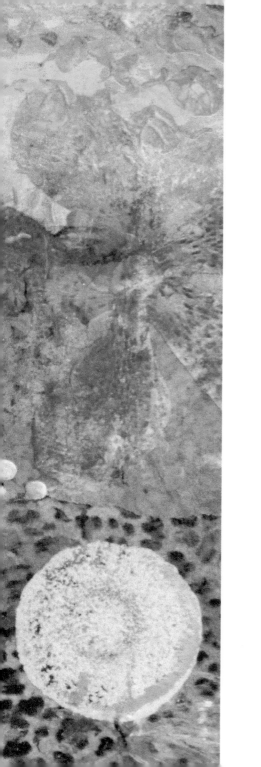

Lightning Source UK Ltd.
Milton Keynes UK
UKOW07f1537111016

285007UK00014B/69/P